Ethics and Nursing Practice

A case study approach

Ruth Chadwick B.Phil., MA, D.Phil., LLB
Director, Centre for Applied Ethics
Philosophy Section
University of Wales College of Cardiff

and

Win Tadd B.Ed.(Hons), DN, RGN, SCM,
ONC, RCNT, Cert.Ed , RNT
Senior Teacher and Project Office⸱ roject 2000
Gwent Health Authority

M
MACMILLAN

First published 1992 by
THE MACMILLAN PRESS LTD
Houndmills, Basingstoke, Hampshire RG21 2XS
and London
Companies and representatives
throughout the world

ISBN 0–333–52045–9

A catalogue record for this book is available
from the British Library.

Printed in Hong Kong

Reprinted 1992 (twice), 1993

Contents

Foreword

One of the special privileges which comes with a request to write the foreword for a book written by someone else is that you are necessarily granted the opportunity to read the manuscript after it has been completed but before its publication. Such a privilege has been mine on several previous occasions. Never has the privilege been as great or the benefits from the preparatory reading so significant as on this occasion.

In the course of my role as a senior member of staff for the statutory body which regulates the nursing, midwifery and health visiting professions in the UK, I meet many practitioners in their respective practice settings, converse with many others when participating in conferences or presenting seminars and respond to the letters and telephone calls of a steadily increasing number. In a majority of such cases the issues that the individual practitioners wish to raise, but have not felt able to raise with colleagues or professional managers in their own settings, are concerned with the ethics of professional practice. Their hesitation to engage in local discussion is usually based on the fact that they are unsure of their ground because, even though they have endeavoured to become informed about ethical principles, if they have found any relevant reading material it has not seemed to address the essentially practical issues which concern them.

I am not intending to suggest that there is a gap in the market for a book that tells the practitioner what to do in a specific set of circumstances. Quite the reverse. Professional practice involves making judgements in a wide variety of circumstances, and being accountable for those judgements.

What I believe to be important, however, is that, before coming face-to-face with a given type of dilemma, practitioners should have had the opportunity to understand and consider the ethical principles that underlie professional practice. One of the most effective ways of doing this is through the use of case studies that provide examples of such dilemmas and open commentary upon them.

I believe that the reader will find, as I have already found, that this book provides not only the means of understanding the theory but of arriving more easily at the solutions to the dilemmas they encounter.

The authors refer, in the opening sentence of their introduction, to the increasing interest in health care ethics. I share their pleasure in that increase and welcome the fact that they have produced such an accessible and informative volume in response to the demand for information that they have identified.

Reginald H. Pyne
Assistant Registrar, Standards and Ethics
United Kingdom Central Council for Nursing Midwifery
and Health Visiting

Acknowledgements

We are indebted to numerous people who, in their various ways, have helped us to write this book. We would first like to thank each and every one of the nurses who shared their experiences of and concerns about nursing practice and without whom this book would not have been possible.

Second, we are grateful to the staff of the Hastings Centre, New York, where, as International Fellows, we were welcomed, encouraged, enabled to research, and involved in lively discussion about many of the issues addressed in this volume.

Although it is not possible to mention everyone at the Centre by name, there are two people in particular who deserve special attention and thanks. Strachan Donnelly, Director of Education, who made our visit possible in the first place and who made lunch-times so memorable. Also, Marna Howarth, Librarian, whose kindness and patience was shown by her tireless assisting with our research, and also on many trips to the supermarket. We shall never forget their help.

Next we would like to thank Dr Lillie Shortridge, Professor and Assistant Dean of Lienhard School of Nursing, Pace University for the time that she devoted to us and her willingness to provide access to postgraduate nurses undertaking a Masters programme.

We are grateful to those nurses on the programme who took time from their studies to provide us with material and, in so doing, brought new dimensions to the book.

Our thanks, too, to Rex Parry and Peter Murby at Macmillan for their advice, understanding and undying patience in the preparation of this volume.

Finally, we would like to thank our partners and families: Stephen Copley for his sense of humour and determination that we should finish; Vic Tadd for his patient reading, helpful comments and endless support and Rebecca and Andrew who were so very understanding when their mother was otherwise engaged.

W.T.
R.F.C.

Introduction

In recent years, there has been increasing interest in health care ethics. Texts, conferences and courses on medical, bio-ethics and indeed nursing ethics are becoming commonplace.

In part, this has been due to advancing scientific and medical technology which has resulted in previously unimaginable treatment possibilities being made available. To a large extent this has resulted in the idea that the ethical issues in health care today are primarily medical and, thus, concern only doctors.

However, this view is being increasingly challenged as professional roles and boundaries are being called into question more often, and because receivers of health care are demanding more involvement in the decisions that often radically affect their lives.

The traditional role of the nurse, as one of exclusively carrying out doctors' orders, is also under scrutiny. Today, many nurses perceive that they have an important role to play in undertaking specific nursing activities, other than those prescribed by medical staff, as well as ensuring that the interests of the patient or client are kept to the fore in all decision-making.

In this volume we hope to show moral principles at work in their application to the sort of real life problems faced by nurses every day. The stimulus for collecting the cases originated from the depth of feeling and concern expressed by many nurses to one of the authors in her work as a nurse teacher.

This led to research, using a critical incident technique, being undertaken with over 400 UK nurses, many of whom were students undertaking pre-registration courses, and some 50 or so qualified nurses undertaking a Master in Nursing course in the USA, to discover the common ethical issues that they faced in their day-to-day practice in the context of today's health care settings.

The point of the exercise is not to say what we, as authors, think about the particular dilemmas. The two of us might not necessarily agree. In some cases the judgement of the writer on a case is made clear, while in others it is not. This in itself is not important. The discussion of the cases is meant to provide a springboard for discussion of the ideas expressed, or a target against which to argue. Nurse teachers may well find the cases useful source material for teaching ethics on both pre- and post-registration courses and individual nurses reading the cases will see how one might approach an ethical dilemma or problem.

Whichever way the book is ultimately used, we hope that it will be of assistance to nurses in tackling the difficult situations which they are likely to face in the course of their work. This may in some small way reduce the tension and stresses that nurses face on an almost daily basis, not only by making their work more rewarding and fulfilling, but also by improving and increasing the quality and humaneness of care afforded to the patient.

The incidents are recounted in the nurses' own words and, again, we are grateful to all those nurses for their willingness that we should publish their stories. Where names of patients are used, these are fictitious to maintain confidentiality.

Some books on nursing ethics begin by presenting a fairly full and detailed exposition of different kinds of ethical theory. We have not taken this approach. Different ethical principles are introduced at various points in the text, and then shown at work in discussing the cases. Suggestions for further reading on ethical theory are provided at the end of the book for those who wish to pursue this further.

Although we do not want to suggest that there is only one 'right' answer to the problems discussed in the book, what we want to stress throughout is the importance of the principle of autonomy. There is a presumption that persons have the capacity to make decisions about their own lives, called a capacity for self-determination or for autonomy. Because of this, the principle of autonomy holds that we should respect the choices that they make (Gillon, 1985, pp. 111–25). This is part of what it means to respect persons.

Because this principle is clearest in the case of the adult, we have discussed the nursing of adults at the beginning of Part II. The adult is called the 'central case' in health care. Even there, as we shall see, there are some problem areas, but the chapters that follow are especially problematic because they deal with groups of patients or clients for whom the presumption of fully developed autonomy does not hold.

The unborn and the newborn, for example, have not yet developed this capacity, so some people argue that they should not be considered as people at all. Children gradually develop their capacity for autonomy, but problems arise about when they become fully autonomous, and to what extent their decisions about treatment should be respected. Persons with a mental handicap or illness suffer from a diminished capacity for autonomy and problems arise about the implications of that for their treatment and care. The person with AIDS still has a capacity for autonomy and is worthy of respect, but this is frequently denied because of the nature of the illness. Elderly people are sometimes thought to have lost, or to be losing their capacity for decision-making, even when there is little evidence to support this in individual cases, which can lead to an unwarranted paternalism – the overriding of their autonomy for what is thought to be their own good. Consideration of those who are terminally ill raises the question of the extent to which persons can retain autonomy, in the sense of control over their own lives, even in their death.

This theme runs through Part II in the discussion of the different groups of clients and patients. In Part I, we stress the importance of the autonomy of the nurse. By this we mean the nurse's capacity to think and decide about the sort of problems covered in this volume. Neither the UKCC Code of Professional Conduct (hereafter referred to as the Code of Conduct) nor other members of the health care team (e.g. senior nurses or doctors) can take away that responsibility. Part I explores the usefulness of guidance such as the Code of Conduct in moral decision-making, and the nurse's relationship with other nurses, the medical profession and the patient or client.

Principles and virtues

As well as the principle of autonomy, there will be discussions about rights, consequences, justice, among other topics. Commonly, there have been two main kinds of ethical theory – roughly, those that appeal to consequences and those which do not. Those that do appeal to consequences proceed by asking 'What will happen if X does this? How will it affect the interests of Y, or the majority of people?' Those that do not, commonly appeal to some set of rules or principles for guidance, and thus avoid the difficulty of trying to predict consequences. The principle of respect for persons, and the view that people have certain rights which must be respected at all costs are of this type. Such non-consequentialist views are commonly classified as 'deontological'. They say what must be done.

The principle of autonomy can be supported by either school, but for different reasons. The non-consequentialists might argue that there is something special about persons that makes them worthy of respect and, as indicated above, to abide by the principle of autonomy is one way of showing respect for persons. The consequentialist, on the other hand, might suggest that it is in the interests of persons to have their autonomous decisions respected, and so it produces the best consequences. One reason for this is that they are quite likely to be the best judges of what is in their own interests, and another is that nothing is more likely to alienate people than having their decisions overruled by those who claim to know better.

It will become clear, however, in the course of the text, that there are several occasions when the interests of different people conflict. Then the person (in our case, the nurse) who has power to affect people's interests has an unenviable task. In such situations, it is difficult to see how it is possible to avoid a consequentialist calculation about how to produce the best result overall. This will involve thinking about the importance of the different interests at stake (some of which may be interests of the nurse) and how to produce the greatest possible satisfaction of interests.

In Chapter 2 we see some of the conflicts between nurses' interests and those of the patient. In this chapter, we also look at a different way of approaching ethics. Instead of discussing principles, we discuss what is known as 'virtue ethics'. Here, the suggestion is that what the good nurse should do is not simply to think about principles, but to acquire certain virtues, such as diligence and candour.

What emerges above all from the cases and the discussion about them is both the extent of and constraints upon the nurse's power to affect standards and ethics in patient care. One reason that we see autonomy as being so central, not only for patients but also for nurses, is that the autonomy of the nurse is vitally important in safeguarding the interests of patients and clients.

The convention used throughout the text, in relation to gender, is that the nurse is referred to as 'she' and others such as the patient or client as 'he', unless the discussion is about an already identified client. This is done only to avoid the use of clumsy he/she references and does not in any way indicate a value belief on the part of the authors, or indeed a lack of awareness of the growing number of male nurses.

With reference to the recipients of health care, both patient and client have been used in recognition of the fact that there is concern on behalf of some nurses to move from the term 'patient' to that of 'client'. We have, therefore, used both terms within the text to take cognisance of this factor.

References

Gillon, R. (1985) 'Autonomy and Consent', in M. Lockwood (ed.), *Moral Dilemmas in Modern Medicine* (Oxford: Oxford University Press).

PART I

PART 1

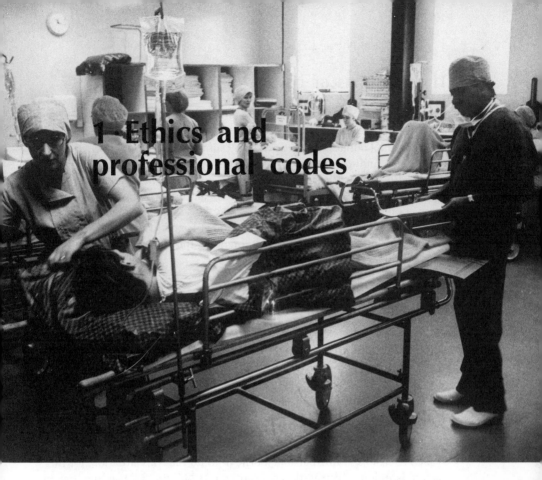

1 Ethics and professional codes

Introduction

In thinking about the principles that nurses might apply when facing moral dilemmas, it is useful to look at the guidance given by professional codes of ethics. In recent years, several codes for nurses have emerged. Not only is there an international code (ICN, 1973), but there are also codes for Canada, the USA, and the UK. In the course of the book we shall be looking at how the UKCC Code of Conduct, in particular, might apply in various situations. Since we are concerned not simply with codes, but with ethics as well, we need to look at how professional codes relate to ethics, and at how useful they are when making moral decisions.

In order to answer these questions, it is necessary to look at what codes are designed to do, and to consider some of the theoretical discussions about their functions. Those readers who prefer to consider more practical issues may wish to miss this section for the time being and to return to it at a later stage, having first seen how clauses of the Code of Conduct relate to moral principles in some of the case studies in this and other chapters of the book.

3

The functions of codes

Competence

Clearly, as Klaidman and Beauchamp point out, one function of codes is to uphold standards of competence, 'even if the word competence is not specifically used in the code' (Klaidman and Beauchamp, 1987, p. 23). But they do more than that. There has been much discussion in recent years about what functions codes perform. It is the task of this chapter to look at various interpretations of their functions and to assess the extent to which codes have a role to play in influencing the ethical decision-making of practitioners.

The ethical function

One possible interpretation, that they provide definitive answers to ethical problems, can be dismissed without too much difficulty. Any list of principles may pose problems for the practitioner, for example when they clash and there is no guidance on priorities, when they are open to different interpretations, or when they simply do not seem to apply to the situation at hand. Thus, Burnard and Chapman, speaking of the UKCC Code of Conduct, say, 'Whilst the Code of Conduct can be used as a guide to such decisions, it must also be borne in mind that this situation, for this person, is unique' (Burnard and Chapman, 1988, p.112). It is significant that Reg Pyne, in his account of the UKCC Code of Conduct, does not mention ethical guidance as one of its defining features (Pyne, 1988, p. 174).

It is also worth noting that the UKCC Code of Conduct is called a Code of Professional Conduct, rather than a code of ethics. The Canadian Code, however, which is a code of ethics, claims that it 'provides clear direction with respect to the avoidance of ethical violations . . . [but] cannot serve the same function for all ethical dilemmas' (CNA, 1985, pp. 1–2). What is being said here is that there are some situations in which our ethical duty is clear; there are some things which must not be done under any circumstances. In less clear cases the Canadian Code attempts to provide guidance only (CNA, 1985, p. 2). But even when there is a situation which the authors of the Canadian Code think is an example of a clear ethical violation, there might be possibilities of disagreement. Veatch and Fry cite the case of a nurse who thought the American Nurses Association (ANA) Code for Nurses was wrong, where her religious beliefs as an orthodox Jew conflicted with the ANA Code's advice that interventions which have the risk of hastening the death of a patient are permissible (Veatch and Fry, 1987, pp. 38–42). Situations such as this lead us to the conclusion that whether or not to abide by the provisions of a code is itself a moral decision (Muyskens, 1982, p. 9).

A code, then, does not resolve ethical dilemmas for a nurse, but it may have considerable influence over her own resolutions to them. In particular, it may stress the most important considerations that should influence a decision. Thus, the UKCC Code of Conduct 'is a statement to the profession of the primacy of the patients' interests' (Pyne, 1988, p. 174).

The political function

Richard Hull suggests that in looking at the function (or functions) of a code we need to examine both its audience and its intent, by a detailed study of the language in which it is written (Hull, 1981, p. 12). The Canadian Code identifies different functions for different audiences. While for new members of the profession it is educative, for established nurses it provides a basis for self-evaluation and peer review (CNA, 1985, p. 1).

The UKCC Code of Conduct does not make these distinctions, stating that all of its provisions apply to every registered nurse, midwife and health visitor, whether newly qualified or senior manager (UKCC, 1984).

However, a code may also be read by members of the public, whether or not they are patients. Then it may provide a means of reassuring them about quality control (Rumbold, 1986, 148–9) or of enhancing the public image of the nurse. In this function its role appears to be political.

Richard Hull identifies this political role of codes as communicatory. They are like a political platform in that they spell out a commitment to a set of ideals. Insofar as they are open to revision they also provide the opportunity for signalling changes in policy (Hull, 1981, p. 12). The ANA Code claims to be 'more a collective expression of nursing conscience and philosophy than a set of external rules' (ANA, 1985, p. iii).

Reg Pyne describes the UKCC Code of Conduct as 'unashamedly political' in that it is a weapon which can be used by nurses to fight for improvements in standards. He says:

> the contents of this code quite deliberately challenge practitioners to become people who challenge. It challenges us to expose risk to patients, where such exists. It challenges us to make demands so that patients and clients receive the standards of care they both need and deserve. It challenges us, if necessary, to adopt a stance which might put us in conflict with people in authority.
>
> (Pyne, 1988, p. 174)

This is a strong statement, which makes it quite clear that the Code of Conduct is not just a piece of window-dressing for the purpose of reassuring the public: it is designed to result in action, action which might sometimes be very difficult for a nurse to take.

Nursing and medical ethics

Another aspect of codes which might be termed political is that they present a picture of what a nurse is, or should be. An early version of the Canadian Code spelled out what was involved in the concept of care (CNA, 1980). Pyne says that the UKCC Code of Conduct points out 'the importance of particular patterns of thought, attitudes, and forms of behaviour' (Pyne, 1988, p. 174). This Code begins with a statement that:

> Each registered nurse, midwife and health visitor shall act at all times in such a manner as to justify public trust and confidence, to uphold and enhance the good standing and reputation of the profession, to serve the interests of society, and above all to safeguard the interests of individual patients and clients.
>
> (UKCC, 1984)

Both the American and the UKCC codes state that each practitioner is accountable for his or her practice (ANA, 1985, s.4.3; UKCC, 1984); Pyne argues that one of the features of the UKCC Code of Conduct is that it is an extended definition of professional accountability (Pyne, 1988, p. 174). The American Code for Nurses explicitly describes the nurse as an advocate for the client (ANA, 1985, s.3.1). The notion of advocacy requires elaboration and will be discussed again in Chapter 2.

In defining the nature of nursing, the codes perform the function of distinguishing nursing from medical ethics. First, as Bandman and Bandman point out, a code reminds nurses and others of the status and importance of nursing in health care (Bandman and Bandman, 1985, p. 36). Further, nursing is portrayed as having specific goals and values which may or may not coincide with those of the medical profession. When they do not, there is the possibility of conflict.

The potential for conflict has been one of the grounds for criticisms of codes for nurses. Hull imagines a patient in hospital trying to find out the extent to which he can expect his confidentiality to be respected. He decides to read the codes for the medical and nursing professions, and finds that they do not entirely coincide in what they say. In this situation, the codes, far from being reassuring, give rise to puzzlement and doubt (Hull, 1980, p. 18).

This problem can only be made worse, argues Hull, if other groups, such as pharmacists and physiotherapists, also have codes of conduct (Hull, 1980, pp. 20–4). Can it really be claimed that their existence is in the best interests of patients? This worry is lessened, however, if codes are seen, not as prescribing how individual members of the profession will behave, but as communicating the goals of the profession.

Professionalism

A further aspect of the political nature of codes for nurses is the role they have to play in supporting professional status. The possession of a code of conduct has been said to be one of the defining characteristics of a profession (Jaggar, quoted in Hull, 1980, p. 19).

The disciplinary function

The relationship of codes to the law may vary according to the particular social context. In the UK, the Code of Conduct was a response to section 2(5) of the Nurses, Midwives and Health Visitors Act 1979, which stated that the UKCC should 'establish and improve standards of training and professional conduct'. Thus, the law gives the Council the power to determine what goes into the Code of Conduct, the contents of which may demand more of a nurse than conformity with the law of the land. Similarly, the ANA Code says that its requirements may often exceed those of the law (ANA, 1985, p. iv).

The requirements of the Code of Conduct are, in the UK, used as 'the backcloth against which allegations of misconduct . . . are now judged' (Pyne, 1988, p. 174). A nurse may lose registration status as a result of a violation of the Code of Conduct, so we may see that it is not simply a guide, nor merely a political document, but also a means of regulating the profession.

Criticisms of codes

Elitism

Hull has pointed out a potential drawback of codes, especially if there is no public participation in their formation. This is that members of the profession may be involved in an elitist enterprise, which carries with it a condescending attitude towards the patients (Hull, 1981, p. 13).

William May makes a similar point in his article 'Code, covenant, contract or philanthropy' (May, 1975). Although he is concerned primarily with codes for the medical profession, his point is a general one, and that is that codes reinforce a view that the professionals are being philanthropic towards the community; that they have certain skills which in their goodness and wisdom they see fit to bestow on those who are in need of them. To take this view, argues May, is to ignore the extent to which the professional group is indebted to the community, both for its education and for the opportunity to practise its skills.

In order to bring out this truth, May suggests that we should not ignore the possibility of basing regulation of the professions on something like a contract with the community, rather than a self-regulatory code (May, 1975).

A contract model is not perfect, however, as May recognises, because if professionals think in terms of a contract they may have little motivation to go beyond the letter of the contract, and may interpret their duties in a minimalist fashion. A code of conduct, as we have seen, makes more stringent demands.

How effective is a code?

Kathleen Fenner makes the point, in relation to the American Code, that it is frequently violated, and puts this down, at least in part, to the fact that nurses are often powerless to control nursing practice (Fenner, 1980, p. 10). She contrasts this with the reasons for the violation of the American Medical Association (AMA) Code, which, she says, tends to be violated because of loyalty to colleagues.

This contrast may be too stark; it is clearly not an easy task to give an account of people's reasons for action. Nevertheless, the point she makes about the nurse's powerlessness is an important one. If nurses are not given sufficient autonomy of action in the hierarchy of the health care setting, this may have a detrimental effect on the standards of care. Fenner points out that nurses often find themselves caught in a conflict between two opposing sets of values: the humanist values which may be reflected in their code, and the authoritarian values of the power structure in which they work (Fenner, 1980, p. 46).

It is in this connection that the importance of Reg Pyne's point becomes clear. If the values of the power structure do conflict with the values of the Code of Conduct, it is the former which must be challenged, but we cannot blind ourselves to the difficulty of this task.

If the Code of Conduct adequately performs its political and educative functions, however, the attitude of and towards nurses will gradually change, and with this their capacity to influence health care. The required change in attitude is partly a question of recognising what power nurses do have. The Canadian Code states that

> Nurses accepting professional employment must ascertain that conditions will permit provision of care consistent with the values and standards of the Code.

> (CNA, 1985, s.VIII)

In the context of a worldwide shortage of nurses, this statement is interesting. If nurses were to abide by it, some quite radical changes could occur in standards of care.

It should be stressed that we are not thinking simply in terms of potential conflict between nurses and the medical profession. Many dilemmas arise from conflicts within the nursing hierarchy itself, and we shall be focusing on these in Chapter 3. The UKCC Code of Conduct quite clearly applies both to nurse managers and to junior staff. Far from being a 'stick' which may be used only by the managers to 'beat' their juniors, the Code of Conduct could be used to point out deficiencies in the manager's standards of care.

The cases

In order to see the role of a code in ethical decision-making, we need to look at some cases. The code to which we shall be referring will be the UKCC Code of Conduct. Within this, it is possible to determine priorities among its various clauses. Since the whole Code of Conduct is a 'statement to the profession of the primacy of the patients' interests' (Pyne, 1988, p. 174), clauses 1 and 2 may be said to take priority. The UKCC has also issued leaflets on some clauses giving guidance as to how they should be interpreted. But, as is stressed in the leaflet on confidentiality, 'the ultimate decision is that of the individual practitioner in the situation' (UKCC, 1987, p. 4). This point has a general application. The Code of Conduct cannot remove from nurses either the capacity or the responsibility to make ethical decisions.

The drug round

❝ I was frightened of her ❞

I was working with the ward sister on an afternoon drug round, and she said, 'I'll bring this patient's medication back later.' The patient confided in me at the end of the shift that he had not received his drugs. During the shift I should have approached the sister but I felt that I ought not to remind her since she was in charge of the ward and partly because I was frightened of her.

Commentary
Many of the cases that come before the UKCC conduct hearings concern inappropriate behaviour in connection with the administering of drugs. The UKCC has issued a leaflet giving guidance for good practice in this area (UKCC, 1986). In the case before us, however, the drugs have not been incorrectly administered: they have not been administered at all. It may seem that this case raises no complicated ethical issues; that the newly qualified nurse should simply have reminded the sister straight out and that that would have been the end of the matter. However, although we may agree that this is what ought to happen, the case is worth

discussing because it illustrates nicely Fenner's point about the reason for many of the violations of nursing codes (Fenner, 1980, p. 10, above). The case-description expresses the difficulty of acting within the context of a power relationship. The nurse feels fear of authority and is insufficiently sure of herself to challenge the ward sister.

If she were to turn to the Code of Conduct what help would it give her? She would see that the fact that the patient had not received his medication was not solely the sister's responsibility. Clause 2 states that the nurse shall 'ensure that no action or omission on his/her part or within his/her sphere of influence is detrimental to the condition or safety of patients/clients'.

In this situation, the condition of the patient was within the nurse's sphere of influence. It was in her power to do something to ensure that he received his drugs and, by doing nothing, she was guilty of an omission to help the patient.

She might, however, look at clause 5, which says that she shall 'work in a collaborative and cooperative manner with other health care professionals and recognise and respect their particular contributions within the health care team'. And as the nurse says of the sister, 'She was in charge'. To be in charge was, arguably, her 'particular contribution'.

As we pointed out earlier, however, the UKCC Code is a statement that the interests of the patient are primary. Clause 1, 'Act always in such a way as to promote and safeguard the wellbeing and interests of patients/clients' is not on an equal footing with clause 5: it takes priority. So, on this interpretation a study of the Code of Conduct should help the nurse to see that where her duty lies is in confronting the ward sister.

We have argued that what a code says can sometimes be at variance with what is morally appropriate behaviour for an individual. In engaging in moral reasoning a nurse is not simply trying to interpret a code in order to find a clear answer to a moral dilemma, but thinking about the reasons behind the statements in that code; the moral considerations and values that support them.

Morally, this case can be read not simply as an issue about the fear of doing the right thing: there is another value at stake, that of respect for authority and hierarchy. This value conflicts with that of concern for the individual patient. The junior nurse feels that it is not up to her to criticise the senior nurse.

What are the arguments, if any, in favour of preserving respect for the authority structure in such a case as this? Many of us are brought up to have respect for authority without thinking very much about it. However, it is part of the task of Ethics to teach us to examine the motives of our actions and to question assumptions that might be deeply ingrained, looking for arguments for or against them.

It might be suggested, in support of authority, that a more efficient service is provided if everyone has a recognised place in the system, associated with certain duties and responsibilities, and that work will run more smoothly as a result. This argument justifies the preservation of the hierarchy in terms of the consequences, or results, it is supposed to achieve, namely, a service which is as efficient as possible in delivering adequate care to patients. But in this case it is clearly not producing the best result, because a patient's interests are being overlooked. So, moral reasoning about the values involved points the same way as the Code of Conduct, namely that the patient's interests are primary, and so must take priority over the preservation of authority structures.

It is clearly a major problem that such structures make it so difficult for nurses to act in the way they feel they ought, and this is something that will be explored further in the chapters on the nurse–doctor relationship and the nurse–nurse relationship (Chapters 3 and 4).

At this point, we shall simply note that the nurse's reading of the Code of Conduct should make it clear to her that it is the sister's duty also to work in a collaborative manner with other members of the team. So she would be in violation of the Code of Conduct if she were to make life difficult for someone who reminded her to do what she should. As Burnard and Chapman say, the value of teamwork lies in its ability to support the novice, while enabling experienced team members to continue learning (Burnard and Chapman, 1988, p. 54).

Confidentiality

❛I get very flushed when I lie❜

After working on a gynaecological ward I met many women who had come in for terminations. Many of these women had told their families that they were in for D&C's or other illnesses. More often than not I was approached by the family or husband and asked for details about the patient. The dilemma was having to lie so frequently. Other staff found the right words, obviously by practice. But unfortunately I get very flushed when I lie, and nearly always make it obvious that I am lying. On one occasion I met one of the women in a local shop with her family. She had become pregnant by a lover, and her family knew nothing of her condition, as she came into hospital for one night while her husband was away. My dilemma was whether to say 'Hello' and risk her husband asking her who I was, or whether to ignore her. The woman looked very nervous, wondering what I was going to say. I chose to give her a discreet smile, but otherwise ignore her. I thought this might save any complications for her.

Commentary
Clause 9 of the Code of Conduct provides that every nurse shall 'respect confidential information obtained in the course of professional practice

and refrain from disclosing such information without the consent of the patient/client . . . except where disclosure is required by law or by the order of a court or is necessary in the public interest'.

In its advisory paper on confidentiality, the UKCC suggests that the focal word in definitions of confidentiality is 'trust', and that where a patient trusts a nurse with confidential information 'the patient/client has a right to believe that this information, given in confidence in the expectation that it will be used only for the purposes for which it was given, will not be released to others without the consent of the patient/client' (UKCC, 1987, p. 6).

In addition to arguments about patients' rights, there are good consequentialist grounds for supporting a principle of confidentiality. If people cannot rely on their confidences being respected, they will be less likely to seek out help when they desperately need it, for problems such as sexually transmitted diseases. Thus, it is not only in the interests of the patient but also in the interests of society generally that people know they can ask advice in confidence.

Both these types of argument for confidentiality, however, come under strain in some circumstances. If we look at rights, it might be argued that one person's right to confidentiality can conflict with another's right to know, or to be protected from harm (e.g. if a patient confides an intention to harm another person). Again, within a consequentialist framework, there may be situations in which it appears that the best consequences will be achieved by disclosing information given in confidence.

The UKCC advisory paper recognises that there will be difficult cases when a patient's interest in confidentiality conflicts with the interest of the public in not being put at risk because practitioners unreasonably withhold information (UKCC, 1987, p. 4). Their position is that the decision in any case is one for the individual practitioner, but one that the practitioner must be able to justify (UKCC, 1987, p. 11). Here, the kinds of argument introduced above would be relevant.

In the case under consideration, it may appear that there are no large issues of the public interest at stake, but there is, nevertheless, a real dilemma for the nurse. When she meets the family in the shop, does she do the correct thing in terms of rights? It is not hard to imagine someone arguing that the husband has a right to know if his wife is having an abortion. Even if this argument is morally sound, there are questions about whether or not it is the nurse's duty to alert him to the facts. For the nurse, the patient's interests are primary, not the husband's.

From a consequentialist point of view, the nurse claims that the decision she took was the one that would be most likely to avoid complications for the woman but, arguably, it is in the best interests of all. When the UKCC refers to 'the dangerous consequences of careless talk in public places' (UKCC, 1987, p. 8), the dangerous consequences can surely include the damage, to all concerned in a relationship, that would be brought about by the disruption of that relationship.

But matters do not end there. Even if we think that the nurse acted appropriately in the shop, she admits that she finds it difficult to cope with this sort of situation on the ward. Is it any more justifiable for nurses to lie to protect patients than it is to lie to protect doctors (cf. Chapter 4)? The fact that she blushes indicates that it is putting the nurse under stress.

Again, any decision is one for the individual practitioner to make and to justify. But, what this case shows us is that there is another set of interests to take into consideration in making that decision, namely the interests of the practitioner herself, and the long-term effects on her of trying to become an accomplished liar. Damage may be limited if patients can find the way to confide in their relatives, or if nurses can find forms of words that do not amount to lies, but there will inevitably be some occasions on which individual nurses have to weigh up one person's interest in confidentiality against the competing interests of others, including her own.

Advertising

> In considering advertising, we shall look at an imaginary case, where a health authority has asked its nurses to wear on their uniforms the logo of a baby food company in exchange for a substantial grant of money towards an increase in neonatal facilities.

Commentary
The UKCC Code of Conduct has a prohibition on advertising. In Clause 14 it states:

> [Each registered nurse shall] avoid the use of professional qualifications in the promotion of commercial products in order not to compromise the independence of professional judgement on which patients/clients rely.

It has been argued that to incorporate a view on advertising brings a code closer to a code of etiquette rather than a code that deals with ethics (Carroll and Humphrey, 1979, p. 24). In other words, it is not morally wrong to advertise, it is simply not 'the done thing'.

Is this view right? Or does the advertising issue raise problems that may correctly be described as ethical ones? In order to assess this, we need to look at the arguments for and against advertising.

Some would argue that advertising is not immoral in itself: it is immoral only if it is dishonest advertising, and any prohibition on nurse advertising should be on the latter only. If we took this view then there would be nothing against those nurses on the unit, who actually did support the products of this particular firm, wearing the company logo on their uniforms. But, on this criterion, it would be wrong for those who believed the products of a rival company to be superior.

From a consequentialist perspective, it might be argued that even those who are opposed to the particular company should wear the logo, on the grounds that it is in the best interests of patients. After all, it will bring in more money for improved facilities, and who will be harmed by it? No-one, in any obvious way.

So what are the arguments against it? First, if a nurse who honestly does not believe in the value of the product wears the logo, she is allowing herself to be used for something about which she disagrees. Even if the advertising is selective, and done only by those nurses who agree with it, there is the danger, as the ANA Code points out, that it 'may be interpreted as reflecting the opinion or judgement of the profession as a whole' (ANA, 1985, s. 10.1). Hence, these nurses may be colluding in the giving of a false impression, however honest their intention. This impression can be foreseen, which is exactly why nurses may prove attractive to commercial companies as potential advertisers. They come into contact with a great many people, when those people are at their most vulnerable and when they are, therefore, likely to develop trust and confidence in their nurses.

Second, there are arguments based on the image of what typifies a nurse. We saw earlier that codes for nurses typically incorporate such an image. If that is incompatible with the suggestion that nurses should be promoting the economic success of particular companies, then no nurse should take part. Thus, the UKCC Code of Professional Conduct points to the importance of 'the independence of professional judgement'.

But what about the view that advertising is in the best interests of patients? We have to think about short-term and long-term interests. To take part in such advertising is a political act – not political in the sense that we argued earlier, that codes are political, but political in the sense that it colludes with the commercialisation of health care generally, rather than promoting the view that health care should be a publicly provided service. This may not be in the best interests of patients in the long-term, if expectations are changed so that units are encouraged to compete for sponsorship in order to be able to provide an adequate service.

It seems, then, that the decision as to whether or not nurses should advertise is indeed an ethical one and, once again, we have seen that ethical reasoning takes us beyond the UKCC Code of Professional Conduct to look at the reasons behind it. A code of conduct or ethics should perhaps be seen, not as the last word on ethics, but as a stimulus to moral thinking.

Conclusion

It is clear that, despite the criticisms that have been levelled against codes, they are useful in providing a stimulus to moral thinking, in promoting the image and interests of the profession and in providing a means of quality control and discipline. As is stressed by the UKCC, however, they cannot replace moral thinking on the part of the individual practitioner. Nurses, like other competent adults, have the capacity for autonomy and for making moral choices, and they do not leave these behind when they go on duty.

The point made in the UKCC advisory paper on confidentiality, that the practitioner must be able to justify decisions taken, shows that ethical practice depends on nurses using their capacity for moral reasoning and autonomous decision-making to think about the Code of Conduct and its application in specific cases. Working conditions, however, may sometimes make this difficult: some problems in this connection will be explored in discussing the nurse–nurse and nurse–doctor relationships (Chapters 3 and 4).

References

American Nurses' Association (ANA) (1985) *Code for Nurses with Interpretive Statements* (Kansas: ANA).

Bandman, E. L. and Bandman, B. (1985) *Nursing Ethics in the Life Span* (Norwalk: Appleton-Century-Crofts).

Burnard, P. and Chapman, C. M. (1988) *Professional and Ethical Issues in Nursing* (Chichester: John Wiley and Sons).

Canadian Nurses Association (CNA) (1980) *CNA Code of Ethics: an Ethical Basis for Nursing in Canada* (Ontario: CNA).

Canadian Nurses' Association (1985) *Code of Ethics for Nursing* (Ontario: CNA).

Carroll, M. A. and Humphrey, R. A. (1979) *Moral Problems in Nursing: Case Studies* (Washington: University Press of America).

Fenner, K. M. (1980) *Ethics and Law in Nursing: Professional Perspectives* (New York: Van Nostrand Reinhold).

Hull, R. T. (1980) 'Defining nursing ethics apart from medical ethics', *Kansas Nurse*, vol. 55, no. 8, pp. 5, 8, 20–4.

Hull, R. T. (1980) 'Codes or no codes?' *Kansas Nurse*, vol. 55, no. 10, pp. 8, 18–19, 21.

Hull, R. T. (1981) 'The function of professional codes of ethics', *Westminster Institute Review*, vol. 1, no. 3, pp. 12–14.

International Council of Nurses (ICN) (1973) *Code of Nursing Ethics* (Geneva: ICN).

Klaidman, S. and Beauchamp, T. L. (1987) *The Virtuous Journalist* (New York: Oxford University Press).

May, W. F. (1975) 'Code, covenant, contract, or philanthropy', *Hastings Center Report*, vol. 5, pp. 29–38.

Muyskens, J. L. (1982) *Moral Problems in Nursing: a Philosophical Investigation* (Totowa: Rowan and Littlefield).

Pyne, R. (1988) 'On being accountable', *Health Visitor*, vol. 61, pp. 173–5.

Rumbold, G. (1986) *Ethics in Nursing Practice* (London: Bailliere Tindall).

United Kingdom Central Council for Nursing, Midwifery and Health Visiting (UKCC) (1984) *Code of Professional Conduct for the Nurse, Midwife and Health Visitor*, 2nd ed. (London: UKCC).

United Kingdom Central Council for Nursing, Midwifery and Health Visiting (UKCC) (1986) *Administration of Medicines* (London: UKCC).

United Kingdom Central Council for Nursing, Midwifery and Health Visiting (UKCC) (1987) *Confidentiality: An Elaboration of Clause 9 of the Second Edition of the UKCC's Code of Professional Conduct for the Nurse, Midwife and Health Visitor* (London: UKCC).

Veatch, R. M. and Fry, S. T. (1987) *Case Studies in Nursing Ethics* (Philadelphia: J. B. Lippincott Co.).

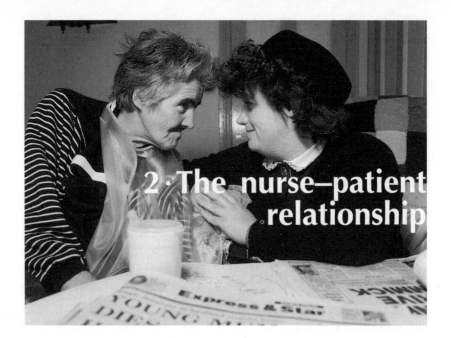

Introduction

The nurse–patient relationship, along with other professional–client relationships, is often described as special (Tschudin, 1986, p. 12). Fromer describes special relationships as 'those in which particular duties and obligations are owed and in which certain duties and obligations go beyond the scope of ordinary social intercourse'. (Fromer, 1981, p. 335).

In Chapter 1, we discussed some of the duties and obligations imposed on nurses by the Code of Conduct (UKCC, 1984). In this chapter, however, we shall explore the nurse's duties, obligations or responsibilities that result from the nurse–patient relationship.

A number of models of nurse–patient relationships have been proposed and it may be helpful to explore at least some of them.

The nurse as parent surrogate

It is undoubtedly this model of the nurse that has significantly influenced nursing and nurse education throughout history (Ashley, 1976, p. 17; Levine, 1977, p. 845). Within such a framework the nurse's responsibility lies in giving care to the patient and acting at all times in the patient's best interests, just as a parent would for a child.

However, not only does this model define the nurse's role, it also defines that of the patient. Dependence is emphasised as is the patient's inability to make decisions, whether this is due to illness, fear, suffering or a reduced capacity for him to understand and appreciate his own needs.

Considerable power is afforded to the nurse for once it is assumed that patients are incapable and dependent, then the nurse can exert extensive influence in decisions regarding their best interests. Any such decisions are most likely to be made from the nurse's value perspective rather than the patient's.

To accept this view of the nurse–patient relationship is to accept nursing as a paternalistic activity. (For discussion of paternalism see Chapter 10.) Some of the case studies discussed in this volume show the frequency with which this role is adopted by nurses in their interactions with patients and clients.

The nurse as technician

Smith (1980, p. 180) proposed this model in response to the view that nursing is primarily a clinical science concerned only with the provision of skilled care which is non-discriminatory, objective and unobtrusive. As Smith points out, the nurse must not impose her values or wishes on the patient but, instead, she must recognise that the patient carries the ultimate responsibility for determining his needs and what is in his own best interests.

Within this model the limit of the nurse's ethical responsibility is the maintenance of competence and the ability to provide skilled care. If the patient requests information then the nurse should give it, but she should not advise the patient as to how best to use it lest, in Gaddow's words, she 'is charged with coercion' (Gadow, 1980, p. 84).

This view of nursing has important consequences for what are widely accepted as appropriate nursing duties. For example, this model would deny any obligation on the part of the nurse to advise clients about health and health related behaviours, unless of course they requested such advice. More importantly, because the nurse's moral values are seen as irrelevant to her role as a nurse, it could be argued that she ceases to be an independent moral agent and merely responds to the patient's bidding.

The nurse as contracted clinician

This model, which was described by Dan Brock (1980), is based on the premise that the patient has the capacity to determine what is in his own best interests and that the ethical duties of the nurse are defined by the patient's rights, chiefly the right to self-determination.

Brock argues that the nurse–patient relationship is based on an agreement or contract between the nurse and the patient. It is the patient who decides not only 'the course of the treatment and care' (Brock, 1980, p. 111), but also the particular role or relationship that the nurse ought to adopt – for example, that of health educator or healer (Brock, 1980, p. 112).

One might be forgiven for asking what then is the difference between the model of the nurse as technician and that of the nurse as contracted clinician? In both instances the patient appears to have the deciding role.

One major difference lies in the importance that is placed on the nurse's moral values. In the technician model these were irrelevant, whereas in a contractual model the nurse can refuse or withdraw from the agreement if her own moral values are compromised.

One criticism that Brock must answer when basing the nurse–patient relationship on the patient's fundamental right to self-determination, is that this right is effectively over-ridden by the fact that the nurse can simply withdraw, thereby allowing the nurse's moral rights to assume priority over the patient's.

A further objection to this account of the nurse–patient relationship is that rarely does any such agreement or contract ever actually take place. Brock's answer to this is that this merely highlights the complexity of modern health care provision rather than showing that the contract model is mistaken.

By accepting health care, the patient makes a general contract to have a variety of services performed by a number of health professionals and the nurse is an indirect party to this agreement by accepting her terms of employment to perform a particular role (Brock, 1980, p. 110).

The problem for the nurse arises when conflicts between her duties to the patient, to the doctor or to the employing institution occur and appeals to the patient's rights offer little help in overcoming such conflicts.

The nurse as patient advocate

The UKCC has stated its expectation that in the exercise of professional accountability 'the practitioner will accept a role as an advocate on behalf of his or her patients/clients' (UKCC, 1989, p. 12). The statutory body goes on to define what, in its opinion, advocacy is and is not. 'Advocacy is concerned with promoting and safeguarding the wellbeing and interests of patients and clients . . . advocacy is a positive constructive activity' (UKCC, 1989, p. 12). '[Advocacy] is not concerned with conflict for its own sake' (UKCC, 1989, p. 12).

It is worth noting that the UKCC does not suggest that advocacy will not involve conflict, merely that it should not do so without reason. Nor does it state which interests and aspects of patient wellbeing should be promoted. Unfortunately, little concrete guidance is given to the nurse who believes that she must take on this mantle.

Any nurse wishing to explore further the concept of advocacy as an acceptable model for professional practice could be excused if she found herself just as bewildered after reviewing the literature that abounds with definitions of what this role would entail.

The following are just a few of those that have been proposed by various authors.

Advocate as counsellor/lay therapist

In this model, the nurse would help to reduce fear, re-establish autonomy and self-control, provide companionship, consolation and attention (Abrams, 1978, p. 260).

Advocate for autonomy

The important element in this definition is that the patient's right to self-determination is absolute. The nurse merely assists the patient to make authentic decisions, that is those that are most in accord with his own values and lifestyles. In no way should the advocate impose or influence the patient in the making of those decisions (Curtin, 1983, p. 9; Abrams, 1978, p. 260; Gadow, 1980, p. 85).

Patient rights advocate

In this case, the nurse would act mainly as a source of information for the patient, advising on legal rights and acting as a watchdog to ensure that such rights are not infringed (Curtin, 1983, p. 9; Abrams, 1978, p. 261).

Advocacy as representation

The function of the nurse in this example is to speak for the patient when he is unable to do so, as for instance when unconscious or incompetent (Abrams, 1978, p. 261).

Advocacy as disinterest or neutrality

This model bears similarities to the nurse as a technician. It emphasises the professional as objective, uninvolved and remote, being there to provide clarification of options and information in a factual or technical manner, but remaining separate from and non-judgemental in the decision-making process (Curtin, 1983, p. 10).

Spiritual advocacy

In this context, the advocate's role is to assist the patient to find unique meaning in his suffering, disability or dying (Gadow, 1980, p. 81).

We need now to consider what each of these models would mean for the nurse–patient relationship although it should be stated that they are not mutually exclusive, nor is the list exhaustive.

Advocacy and the nurse–patient relationship

The first two models are proposed because the nurse enjoys close and continuing patient contact and therefore is in an ideal position to perform such functions, but dangers also exist because of the nurse's intimate and close contact with patients.

The patient, because of illness, is to a large extent dependent upon the nurse: first, in a physical sense which often involves the nurse in performing very intimate procedures and, second, emotionally dependent due to fear, pain or separation from family and friends.

The patient has little control of the situation as he cannot withdraw and, therefore, the nurse occupies a powerful position in relation to the patient who is very vulnerable to both coercion and persuasion.

A further problem involving the first model is that most nurses do not possess the skills or knowledge to enable them to function competently as counsellors and there are dangers in encouraging them to believe that they can (Abrams, 1978, p. 262).

A major difficulty with the second model, highlighted by Curtin (1983, p. 10), is that it could be seen to deny professional responsibility and accountability by defining advocacy as promoting the patient's self interest.

What does this account of advocacy mean for the nurse who works with individuals who are dependent upon alcohol or drugs? Such individuals may well believe that the continued use of these substances is in their best interests. Does this impose on the nurse a duty to obtain alcohol or drugs for them or at least to turn a blind eye when patients persist in taking them?

Obviously, any nurse taking such actions would be deemed irresponsible, if not condemned for being unprofessional. So, advocacy based exclusively on the promotion of patient autonomy, when this is defined as the right to self-determination, ought to be rejected.

The major problem with the nurse acting as patient rights advocate is the lack of knowledge that most nurses possess with regard to the law and its application in particular circumstances. This could, of course, be remedied by extending nurse education to include a significant amount of legal content, but would this totally resolve the difficulties?

If we consider this alongside the fourth model of advocacy as representation then the difficulties of acting in another's interest are readily apparent.

Curtin (1983, p. 9) recounts an incident in which a nurse anaesthetist refused to administer an anaesthetic to a patient who was refusing to have a pacemaker inserted, asserting that this would override the patient's legal right to refuse treatment. The woman was in a rapid atrial fibrillation which could not be controlled by any alternative treatment.

The family, the attending doctor and the nurses in the coronary care unit, where the patient was being nursed, decided that the woman's condition had deteriorated to such an extent that a pacemaker had to be inserted. They pointed out that cerebral hypoxia due to the reduced cardiac output might explain why this patient refused to give consent.

A second nurse was found who was willing to administer anaesthesia, and the pacemaker was successfully inserted. The woman was restored to near normal life and could not remember refusing to give consent.

Curtin quite rightly asks which nurse acted as patient advocate? Not only do patients have the legal right to refuse treatment, but they also have a right to receive treatment. Nurses, as well as other health care professionals, have a duty to provide it, especially when the patient's condition is such that it can detract from that right. In other words, to ensure that the patient's best interests are represented.

Patients' rights are often in conflict with one another as in this case when the right to refuse treatment could have conflicted with the right to life itself. The difficulty in such cases is whether the advocate should speak for the patient as the first nurse did or act to safeguard the patient's life as those recommending the surgery did. Another way of posing this question would be to ask to what extent is paternalistic action justified?

This notion of advocacy, as either defender of patient rights or as patient representative, also appears to be fraught with difficulty and contradiction.

When we consider advocacy as disinterest or neutrality even more problems emerge. Most members of the public seek professional advice because the professional has expertise in a particular area. Imagine consulting a solicitor and, after having various options outlined without any of the ensuing implications, being told to make our own decisions as to which was the best.

Surely we would consider this very strange as part of the reason for seeking the consultation in the first place is to hear what the expert thinks.

The public expect that those involved in health care do actually care about the wellbeing of individual patients and to force people to make decisions in isolation seems callous at the very least.

In criticising spiritual advocacy, Curtin suggests that to seek to explain why certain individuals have been singled out for disease or suffering is nothing short of cruel and destructive. The appropriate role for the nurse is to provide comfort and reduce suffering rather than to explore its meaning for the individual concerned (Curtin, 1983, p. 9).

There are other general criticisms of advocacy as an appropriate role for the nurse. First, unlike the situation with other professionals who adopt this role, such as lawyers, the patient is unable to choose his nurse and therefore his advocate. This presents great difficulties, especially if one judges advocacy to be representation.

Second, nurses rarely have only one patient's interests to consider, and advocacy can pose problems when interests between patients conflict, particularly in long-stay residential settings where this is likely to happen.

Third, who will act for the patient when an advocate is needed *against* the nurse, for nurses can be just as fallible as other health professionals.

Fourth, how is the nurse to answer challenges from other health care professionals who believe that they too act as patient advocates. To do this successfully the nurse needs to be able to show that she has the requisite skills and knowledge to perform this role adequately.

Finally, successful advocacy on behalf of patients would best be undertaken by an independent agent who is free of institutional and other constraints.

The greatest problem for the nurse in adopting this role lies in the fact that she has obligations other than those to the patient. She has obligations to medical staff to carry out prescribed treatments, to the institution that employs her and to senior nursing staff to act in accordance with agreed nursing policy and procedures.

How the nurse is to balance these obligations is not clear. Merely to assert that the nurse adopt the role of advocate, without specific guidance, could be viewed as unethical as this places her in a very vulnerable position.

In the USA Corrine Warthen was dismissed by her hospital following refusal to carry out further dialysis on a terminally ill patient. The patient, on two previous occasions of dialysis, had suffered cardiac arrest and severe internal haemorrhaging (Warthen vs. Toms River Community Memorial Hospital, 1985, pp. 229–234).

Warthen, after asking not to be assigned to the patient again, refused to dialyse the patient on moral, philosophical and medical grounds and in accordance with the American Nurses Association Code of Conduct. Clause 3 of this document states that, 'The nurse acts to safeguard the client and the public when health care and safety are affected by incompetent, unethical or illegal practice of any person' (ANA, 1985).

This statement concurs with the UKCC's notion of advocacy as being 'concerned with promoting and safeguarding the wellbeing and interests of patients'. So, Ms Warthen could clearly have perceived herself to be acting as patient advocate.

Warthen, believing that she had been wrongfully dismissed, took her case to the Supreme Court. Unfortunately, the New Jersey court ruled that the ANA Code was not a statement of public policy, but rather 'a standard of conduct beneficial only to the nurse.' (Blum, 1984, p. 150). Warthen's dismissal was accordingly deemed fair.

This case illustrates the problems that arise, due to the conflicting loyalties experienced by the nurse, in giving patient care. Also, the statutory body offers little help when encouraging advocacy by merely stating that 'Each practitioner must determine exactly how this aspect of personal professional accountability is satisfied within her particular sphere of practice' (UKCC, 1989, p. 12).

Advocacy appears to offer confusion and considerable risk to nurses and perhaps in the words of Kath Melia, it is 'one bandwagon that nurses should let pass by' (Melia, 1989, p. 38).

A relationship of trust

The search for a single ideal model for the nurse–patient relationship appears to resemble the search for the Holy Grail and this is hardly surprising when one considers that relationships are rarely static. They develop and change in accordance with their function and the nurse–patient relationship is no exception. One would hardly expect the relationship between a nurse and a newly admitted patient, who is critically ill following a myocardial infarction, to remain unaltered up to the moment of discharge.

For one thing the patient's physical and emotional needs will have changed, as will the nurse's knowledge of the patient as a person, and to a large extent both of these factors will inform the developing relationship.

One factor which ought to remain constant throughout the encounter is that the patient can trust the nurse, hence the use of the term fiduciary in describing any client/professional relationship.

It may be that our time could be more profitably spent in considering what general obligations are placed on the professional because of this special trust that most clients have.

Michael Bayles identifies six obligations which professionals owe to clients if they are to be deserving of their trust (Bayles, 1981, p. 71).

Honesty

The opening statement of the Code of Conduct commences as follows:

> Each registered nurse, midwife, and health visitor shall act, at all times, in such a manner as to justify public trust and confidence, to uphold and enhance the good standing and reputation of the profession.
>
> (UKCC, 1984, p. 2)

Clearly professionals have no automatic right to expect the public to place their trust in them. Instead, it has to be earned and nurses are no different from any other professional in this respect. To warrant such belief, certain standards of behaviour are expected of people occupying particular positions in society.

Nurses are often in a privileged position in relation to patients' money, valuables or property as the following examples show. District nurses, midwives and health visitors enter private houses on a daily basis. Nurses working in accident and emergency departments handle patients' valuables and money, often without the knowledge of the patients themselves. Nurses working with long-stay clients, such as those that are elderly, mentally ill or mentally handicapped, frequently take groups of residents on outings and holidays which often involves them in handling large sums of spending money belonging to the patients.

Clause 8 of the Code of Conduct recognises the potential for dishonesty and demands that members of the profession 'avoid any abuse of the privileged relationship which exists with patients/clients and of the privileged access allowed to their property, residence or workplace' (UKCC, 1984, p. 3).

Honesty is an essential attribute in the nurse and for this reason nurses are not exempt under the Rehabilitation of Offenders Act. This means that they must declare any criminal prosecutions and unlike other members of the public, convictions are never spent.

Candour

Bayles, (1981, p. 72) describes candour as a subclass of honesty. It is concerned with truthfulness, although it demands more than the avoidance of lying. For example, it is possible to avoid lying by refraining from answering a question, but this would involve a lack of candour which requires full disclosure or the absence of deceit.

The trust which exists in the nurse–patient relationship makes truthfulness extremely important, and the UKCC document *Exercising Accountability* emphasises the problems that can result when practitioners are economical with the truth, 'the damage to public trust and confidence in the profession . . . will be enormous' (UKCC, 1989, p. 11).

By withholding information when it is sought by the patient, the nurse is showing a lack of respect for the client's judgement and manipulating his actions thereby changing the fiduciary nature of the nurse–patient relationship to one of paternalism.

There are many reasons why nurses may decide to be less than candid with patients. The patient may have requested not to be informed of a poor or disturbing diagnosis and, in such instances, his wishes ought to be respected. However, other reasons may be less altruistic.

Sometimes, it is the easy option in that it saves a great deal of distress for the nurse as well as the patient. A doctor or senior nurse may decide that to tell the whole truth will cause 'harm' to the patient and this poses problems for junior members of the team who are then ordered not to disclose. Harm is a slippery concept which involves complex value judgements made on behalf of someone else. Psychological distress may, in some instances, be classed as harm but the distress caused by the knowledge of a poor prognosis may be short-lived when compared with the effects, on the individual and his family and friends, of living a lie.

Competence

A public expectation of professionals is that they are competent to fulfil the service that they offer. Although competence is not a moral attribute, for a professional to pretend to be competent when she isn't, is a betrayal of public trust in her ability.

Current debate in the UK on the subject of mandatory updating is evidence of the importance placed on this aspect of the nurse's role. Regardless of how that particular debate continues, two clauses of the Code of Conduct are concerned with this professional responsibility.

Clause 3 states that the individual practitioner must, 'Take every reasonable opportunity to maintain and improve professional knowledge and competence' (UKCC, 1984, p. 2).

This means that it is not enough for the nurse to merely arrive on duty, complete her shift to the best of her ability and go home. A moral obligation is placed on each individual to read professional journals, to update their knowledge and, of course, to implement well researched improvements in nursing care.

There is, however, another aspect of competence which imposes further responsibilities on the nurse, and this is highlighted in clause 4 which states that the nurse, midwife and health visitor must:

> Acknowledge any limitations of competence and refuse in such
> cases to accept delegated functions without first having received
> instruction in regard to those functions and having been assessed
> as competent.

> (UKCC, 1984, p. 2)

This, to a large extent, may be seen to refer to what is regarded as the 'extended role of the nurse' and may cover such duties as giving intravenous injections or performing defibrillation in emergency situations. Clearly, it would be extremely dangerous for a nurse to undertake these functions without adequate preparation.

However, as nurses progress through their careers it is all too easy to lose the ability to perform nursing skills with the same dexterity as when these were practised on a daily basis. Similarly, certain areas of knowledge become outdated, for example new drugs come onto the market almost weekly.

Nurses, whose current roles take them out of daily clinical practice, must therefore exercise caution when, infrequently, they find themselves involved in direct patient care. Nurse managers and teachers may constitute two such groups and much has been written recently regarding joint appointments or lecturer/practitioner roles which enable teachers to maintain clinical competence while fulfilling their responsibilities for teaching. Indeed, one might wish to argue that if one is teaching or managing a practice based discipline, such as nursing, then one has a moral obligation to remain clinically competent.

Diligence

Diligence requires more than competence. It requires commitment and attention. Claims for negligence are often the result of a lack of diligence which causes an adverse outcome for a patient or client which, had more care been exercised, could have been avoided.

Iris Murdoch differentiates between the neutrality of 'looking' and the moral nature of 'seeing' by incorporating the need for attention in seeing. 'The moral sense of 'see' which implies that clear vision is a result of moral imagination and moral effort' (Murdoch, 1970, p. 37).

In other words, it is often the case that one sees what one expects to see, rather than what is actually there. A commitment to care requires the additional effort of looking to ensure that what one sees is indeed what is there.

Nurses frequently claim that they are too busy to 'see' or be diligent, hence the large numbers of drug errors which occur. The Code of Conduct places a professional obligation on the nurse to ensure that workloads are such that they do not 'constitute abuse of the individual practitioner . . . or jeopardise safe standards of practice' (UKCC, 1984, p. 3).

This poses a dilemma especially for the nurse manager who must then decide whether the pressures are such that she must close beds, thereby denying services to patients not yet admitted, in order to provide diligent care to existing patients.

Nursing has a tradition of coping no matter how difficult the situation is and perhaps today more than ever before, with increasing restrictions on resource allocation, it is time for nurses to recognise that professionalism brings with it a demand for political activity.

Nurses have obligations to potential patients as well as those in existence and, therefore, they have a duty in the public interest to bring to attention, conditions which militate against safe standards of care (UKCC, 1989, p. 9).

Loyalty

Loyalty has been a traditional value throughout nursing's history and a great deal has been written about how this could be best achieved (Percy and Kirkpatrick, 1917, p. 24; Davis and Aroksar, 1978, pp. 12–13; Aikens, 1916, p. 44). Gerald Winslow suggests that the concept of loyalty was largely concerned with 'the protection of confidence in the health care effort' (Winslow, 1984, p. 33).

Translated into daily practice this meant that, as well as being faithful to the patient, the nurse should not criticise the institution in which she was employed, her teachers and colleagues, or indeed the medical staff whose orders she had to follow.

Loyalty to the physician is an issue which we shall explore in detail in Chapter 4, but it is interesting to note that loyalty to the patient was interpreted as showing loyalty to the doctor. 'Loyalty to the physician and faithfulness to the patient do not form a twofold purpose, but a single one' (Satterthwaite, 1910, p. 109).

The conflicting loyalties which nurses still face (Rhodes, 1983, pp. 65–6; Copp, 1988, pp. 42–4), raise issues not only of professional autonomy, but also of personal interest conflicting with patient interest.

The Code of Conduct (clause 5) demands collaboration and cooperation of nurses in respect of their work with other health professionals (UKCC, 1984, p. 2). However, in its later document *Exercising Accountability*, the statutory body also recognises the clash of interests that can occur in multidisciplinary working and it advises that 'in such circumstances it is important to stress that the interests of the patient or client must remain paramount' (UKCC, 1989, p. 14).

To be loyal the nurse must, in balancing her multiple obligations, be careful to ensure that loyalty to the patient remains a priority. This requires the use of independent judgement and a degree of objectivity in professional decision-making, as well as courage to exercise both moral and professional autonomy.

Discretion

The final attribute that Bayles recommends in the professional/client relationship is that of discretion. He differentiates this from confidentiality by describing it as a broader concept which embraces material which is not of a confidential nature (Bayles, 1981, p. 83).

Being discreet in our interactions with others is part of the principle of respect for persons in that it recognises their right to privacy. Providing nursing care frequently involves the nurse in undertaking intimate actions on behalf of patients that would ordinarily be fulfilled in privacy. For example, hygiene and elimination needs are not usually met under the eye of a total stranger, just as showing extreme distress in public is not a social norm in our culture.

The nurse is directly involved in such patient care situations on a daily basis and it would be wrong to betray the patient's trust by causing embarrassment through ridicule or indiscreet gossip with other nurses or patients.

Nursing as caring

Nursing is often described as a 'caring profession' and it may be worthwhile to consider the implications for caring from the foregoing.

To care for another person involves understanding them in their own situation, namely showing empathy as opposed to sympathy. The difficulty with expressing sympathy is that there is a danger of the nurse becoming so involved on the patient's problem that she risks losing her own identity.

Mayerhoff emphasises this need for objectivity in caring to enable the carer to be aware of her own reactions to the situation in which the one being cared for finds himself. For example the nurse does not have to *be* anxious to appreciate the anxiety that the patient experiences, but by appreciating it, she is in a better position to relieve the patient's worries (Mayerhoff, 1972, p. 42).

Caring requires that the nurse sees the patient as an equal in the relationship. This should not be in terms of knowledge and expertise, but as a person equally deserving of respect, and so she must deliver care in a non-judgemental way that will not diminish the patient as a person.

The nurse needs to recognise that it is important not only for the patient to trust her but also that she must trust the patient. In doing so, she recognises his autonomy and promotes his independence. By always doing things and making decisions for the patient, the nurse is maintaining his dependence and denying both the need and opportunity for him to take responsibility.

Caring demands patience: time and willingness on behalf of the nurse to come to know the patient as a person and to better understand his needs. It may also demand moral courage to ensure that the focus of care is the primacy of the patient's interest. Finally, it demands commitment on the part of the nurse, that is the willingness to undertake actions to the very best of one's ability, not merely because one has to, but because one wants to do so.

The cases

Ignoring a patient

❛I have felt guilty ever since❜

I had had a hard day on a busy ward and hadn't been able to do anything right. I was already fifteen minutes late when Sister said I could go. Just then I heard a patient ask for help to go to the toilet.

I ignored the patient and went home. I have felt guilty ever since and now I would never leave a patient in need, no matter what the time was.

Commentary

This case raises the role of conscience in moral decision-making. Although this has been much discussed in moral philosophy, it may be worthwhile spending a short time exploring this concept in relation to the nurse.

If one were to ask friends or colleagues why they chose a particular course of action they would frequently reply that their conscience had guided them. But what is conscience?

Beauchamp and Childress define conscience as 'a mode of thought about one's acts and their rightness or wrongness, goodness or badness' (Beauchamp and Childress, 1983, p. 270). Some philosophers, such as Bishop Butler (1967), held that the individual's conscience was the ultimate authority in determining right or wrong actions and today many individuals believe that, when confronted by an ethical dilemma, their conscience will provide them with the ultimate guidance. But is this belief in conscience justified?

One of the problems with the concept of individual conscience is that not everyone's conscience gives the same direction. People can justify a variety of very questionable behaviours on the grounds that they acted in accordance with their conscience. Eichmann was one such example.

The individual's conscience is personal and tends to be a reflective judgement of his actions against personally held moral standards, hence the oft' heard remark that 'I could not live with myself if I did such and such'. In other words, we have already decided that a particular act is wrong and if we go ahead and perform the act, then our conscience nags us and we experience a sense of guilt.

The debate as to whether these moral standards are rationally derived or are a result of our early socialisation, as Freud suggests, continues to flourish but clearly conscience itself does not determine what is in fact right or wrong.

In the case described, it is not clear whether there were pressing reasons, other than tiredness and feelings of frustration, why the nurse should overrule the dictates of her conscience. It may have been that someone was waiting for her or that she had family commitments to fulfil after her day's work.

Indeed, had she answered the patient's call for help she may have been so tired that she could have endangered the patient's safety. Or, feeling resentful, she may have displayed anger or annoyance toward the patient thereby damaging his self-esteem. Either of these consequences could have been far worse than waiting a few moments for the next nurse coming on duty.

Furthermore, there is a limit as to how long a nurse ought to remain on duty after completing a full day. What if after helping this patient another had asked for help. Considering the principle of justice, is it fair to the nurse to expect her to go on answering patient requests? How do we decide which patient to respond to when there are a number whose needs are unmet at the end of a span of duty?

In other words, guilt can often be misplaced. Although we might view the situation differently had the patient been bleeding to death, on the face of it, it appears that this nurse is judging herself very harshly.

The case does highlight another serious limitation to using conscience as the only guide to moral actions. That is, when it is in our own interest, it can be very easy to ignore the call of conscience and give in to other desires.

This nurse could perhaps learn better from the experience if she considered which moral principle she overruled in ignoring the patient. For example, beneficence and how it might have been possible for her to both act in the patient's interest and satisfy her own need to go off duty. This could have been achieved by informing the nurse coming on duty that the patient needed help to go to the toilet.

Reflecting on one's moral actions with a view to finding morally acceptable alternatives is a more positive approach to determining future behaviour than either subjecting oneself to pangs of guilt or to setting standards which will be impossible to reach.

The use of placebos

❝ She was furious that we had deceived her ❞

Emma was a 52-year-old woman who had suffered chronic back pain for many years. She had had repeated admissions in an attempt to find the cause, all without success, and her only relief came from the Pentazocine which she had taken for years.

Along with the doctors, Sister agreed that sterile water should be given as a substitute without Emma's knowledge, as it was believed that Emma was so addicted that it was difficult to know whether she really had pain or not.

Gradually all of Emma's analgesia was replaced with the water, despite her complaints of cramps, nausea and pain. After a few weeks she was told that her drugs had been substituted and that it was now possible to control her pain with a milder and safer analgesic.

She was furious that we had deceived her and accused us of causing her unnecessary suffering. When she left the ward she vowed that she would never return to the hospital.

Sister felt that the actions were justified as Emma would have a better life free from the drug.

Commentary

The moral issue raised by this case is whether or not a nurse is justified in participating in this type of deception that the use of placebos necessitates.

It is not clear whether less deceptive means to reduce this patient's dependence were attempted and failed or because of expedience were never tried. If one agrees that candour and trust are important aspects of the nurse–patient relationship, then it is difficult to see how such action might be judged as appropriate, as it denies patient autonomy and the right to participate in decision-making about modifying one's own life-style.

The sister in this case might have argued that Emma's autonomy was already impaired because of either addiction to the drug or extreme fear of pain should she discontinue its use. One needs to exercise caution, however, as claims of impaired autonomy can be used by professionals to ensure that their goals, rather than the patient's, are met. The sister needs to ask herself whether she would have still believed that Emma's autonomy was impaired if she had agreed to dispense with the drug voluntarily.

The major objection to such practices is the damage to the trust that patients inevitably invest in health professionals when such deception is ultimately discovered. Sissela Bok highlights this danger when she states

> the practice of giving placebos is wasteful of a very precious good: the trust on which so much in the medical relationship depends. The trust of those patients who find out that they have been duped is lost, sometimes irretrievably.

(Bok, 1978, p. 63)

The fact that this patient vowed never to return to the hospital appears to indicate that she had lost faith in the staff. This loss of faith and trust not only involves the doctors and the sister, but probably all of the nurses who had given her injections of sterile water. As Bok goes on to point out, such a loss of trust could result in patients not seeking professional help in the event of future illness (Bok, 1978, p. 63).

A second justification for this type of deception is the one that the sister alludes to, namely that the ends justify the means. In other words, Emma is freed from her addiction to the drug and her pain can be controlled by less potent drugs.

This is another form of paternalistic behaviour which involves deception as a form of manipulation or coercion to ensure that another person behaves in the way that one wants them to. Regardless of the benevolent motives which might prompt such behaviour, it undermines the rights of the individual to be treated as a person, as their values, choices and desires are disregarded.

Immanuel Kant, an 18th century philosopher who wrote at length about respect, would have determined that such actions are contrary to his second formulation of the categorical imperative that one should 'Act in such a way that you always treat humanity whether in your own person or in the person of any other, never simply as a means, but always at the same time as an end' (Kant, 1956, p. 96).

Despite the fact that the outcomes of this patient's management were satisfactory, nurses need to be aware that the use of such 'ends justify the means' arguments can lead to very questionable moral practices and, therefore, they should be used only as a last resort after non-deceptive means have been tried.

Punishing patients

❮ *She was always moaning at the nurses* ❯

A senior staff nurse refused to help me lift a patient out of the bath saying that she was always moaning at the nurses and that it might do her good to stay there. Consequently the patient remained in the bath for 35 minutes and despite my efforts to keep running warm water, the patient became very cold.

Eventually, an auxiliary helped me to return the patient to her bed. I reported the incident to sister, but no action was taken. As there were only two of us on duty at the time and the patient was very overweight, it would have been very dangerous for me to attempt to lift her out on my own.

Commentary

Labelling people is as commonplace in nursing as it is in other social interactions. For example, patients may be described according to their abilities such as 'ambulant' or 'dependant' or according to the nature of their particular treatment, such as 'medical' or 'surgical'. Categorising or making generalisations about people and objects is one of the first things that young children learn to do, but not all labelling is as harmless as that described above.

Labelling is frequently used to reflect one's perceptions of and attitudes towards individuals who in one way or another deviate from the expected norms of a particular culture. Once a patient becomes labelled as 'awkward' or 'difficult' then nursing staff come to expect and indeed look for instances of behaviour that justify the label.

Another effect of labelling is that nurses can use the label to justify the feelings, attitudes and behaviours that they display towards patients. The staff nurse in this case justified leaving the patient in the bath because she was always moaning.

Once labelled, any behaviour displayed by the person is attributed to their disposition rather than to the situation, and this is termed the fundamental attribution error (Hilgard et al, 1979, p. 543). This patient's continued 'moaning' is seen as a feature of her personality. However, it is conceivable that, with staff as uncaring as this particular nurse appears to be, the patient may have been justified in making her dissatisfaction known.

This highlights quite clearly that the expectation of some nurses is that complaining is not a legitimate activity for someone cast in the role of patient, but instead it is assumed that they ought to be grateful for the care that they receive.

Having labelled this patient as ungrateful, the staff nurse appears to be punishing her, but is punishment an appropriate or acceptable solution?

Punishment necessarily involves deliberate harm which may be justified on the grounds of 'just desert', retribution or reforming the offender. In this case, the patient became chilled, her skin could have been adversely affected and presumably she was distressed by the incident. It seems unlikely that punishment of this nature would reform the patient, rather it is likely to bring further complaints and so is the staff nurse attempting to exact retribution?

That some nurses may feel it is appropriate to 'get their own back' in this way is somewhat alarming as it smacks of controlling patients in a way that abuses the nurse–patient relationship. Patients, regardless of their condition, are vulnerable and often extremely stressed. This places the onus on the nurse to control her own feelings however understandably negative they may be, and treat patients with kindness and courtesy.

This does not mean that the patient's apparent dissatisfaction cannot be openly and honestly discussed. This in itself may resolve the problem if the patient recognises that her demands are unrealistic.

One of the most disturbing aspects of this case is to be found in the last paragraph. This nurse had the courage to report the unsatisfactory treatment of a patient by a member of the nursing team and it appears that no action was taken. The basis of the nurse–patient relationship, as we have already seen, is one of trust and providing care. The failure to take action to maintain and improve standards is not only an abuse of that trust, but it may result in nurses becoming apathetic about reporting such incidents to the detriment of patients and the profession alike.

Conclusion

This chapter has focused on a variety of models that have been proposed for the nurse–patient relationship as well as some of the obligations that are incumbent on individual nurses involved in caring. From these considerations, we have seen that trust is essential if nursing is to be a moral endeavour.

The first case demonstrated the unrealistic expectations that nurses, or perhaps their early socialisation into the profession, place upon themselves, as well as the dangers of using conscience as the ultimate guide to morality.

The last two cases highlighted the ways that trust can be abused not only in relation to patients but also other nurses, and the consequences that can result from such abuse.

References

Abrams, N. (1978) 'A Contrary View of the Nurse as Patient Advocate', *Nursing Forum*, vol. XVII, pp. 258–59.

Aikens, C. A. (1916) *Studies in Ethics for Nurses*, p. 44 (Philadelphia: W. B. Saunders).

American Nurses Association (1985) *Code for Nurses with Interpretive Statements* (Kansas City: ANA).

Ashley, J. A. (1976) *Hospitals, Paternalism and the Role of the Nurse*, p. 17 (New York: Teachers College Press).

Bayles, M. D. (1981) *Professional Ethics*, pp. 70–86 (Belmont: Wadsworth Publishing Company).

Beauchamp, T. L. and Childress, J. F. (1983) *Principles of Biomedical Ethics*, 2nd ed., p. 270 (New York: Oxford University Press).

Blum, J. D. (1984) 'The Code for Nurses and Wrongful Discharge', *Nursing Forum*, vol. 21, p. 150.

Bok, S. (1978) *Lying* (London: Quartet Books Limited).

Brock, D. (1980) 'The Nurse–Patient Relation: Some Rights and Duties', in S. F. Spicker and S. Gaddow (eds), *Nursing Images and Ideals: Opening Dialogue with the Humanities* (New York: Springer Publishing Company).

Butler, J. (1967) 'Sermons', in A. I. Melden (ed.), *Ethical Theories: a book of readings*, 2nd ed. (Englewood Cliffs, NJ: Prentice-Hall).

Copp, G. (1988) 'Professional Accountability: The Conflict', *Nursing Times*, vol. 84, no. 43, pp. 42–4.

Curtin, L. L. (1983) 'The nurse as advocate: a cantankerous critique, *Nursing Management*, vol. 14, May, pp. 9–10.

Davis, A. J. and Aroskar, M. A. (1978) *Ethical Dilemmas and Nursing Practice* (New York: Appleton Century Crofts).

Fromer, M. J. (1981) *Ethical Issues in Health Care* (St. Louis: C. V. Mosby).

Gadow, S. (1980) 'Existential Advocacy: Philosophical Foundation of Nursing', in S. F. Spicker and S. Gaddow (eds), *Nursing Images and Ideals: Opening Dialogue with the Humanities* (New York: Springer Publishing Company).

Hilgard, E. R., Atkinson, R. L. and Atkinson, R. C. (1979) *Introduction to Psychology*, 7th ed. (New York: Harcourt Brace Jovanovich).

Kant, I. (1956) *Groundwork of the Metaphysic of Morals*, 3rd ed., translated by H. J. Paton (New York: Harper and Row).

Levine, M. E. (1977) 'Nursing Ethics and the Ethical Nurse', *American Journal of Nursing*, May, p. 845.

Mayerhoff, M. (1972) *On Caring* (New York: Harper and Row).

Melia, K. (1989) *Everyday Nursing Ethics* (Basingstoke: Macmillan).

Murdoch, I. (1970) *The Sovereignty of Good* (Bristol: Routledge and Kegan Paul).

Percy, T. and Kirkpatrick, C. (1917) *Nursing Ethics* (Dublin: Dublin University Press).

Rhodes, B. (1983) 'Accountability in Nursing: Alternative Perspectives', *Nursing Times*, Sept. 7, pp. 65–6.

Satterthwaite, T. E. (1910) 'Private Nurses and Nursing: With Recommendations for their Betterment', *New York Medical Journal*, vol. 91, p. 109.

Smith, S. (1980) Three models of 'The nurse–patient relationship', in S. F. Spicker and S. Gaddow (eds), *Nursing Images and Ideals: Opening Dialogue with the Humanities* (New York: Springer Publishing Co.).

Tschudin, V. (1986) *Ethics in Nursing: The Caring Relationship* (London: Heinemann).

United Kingdom Central Council for Nurses, Midwives and Health Visitors (1984) *Code of Professional Conduct*, 2nd ed. (London: UKCC).

United Kingdom Central Council for Nurses, Midwives and Health Visitors (1989) *Exercising Accountability* (London: UKCC).

Warthen vs. Toms River Community Memorial Hospital, Supreme Court of New Jersey, AD, 8/1/85–14/2/82 in *Atlantic Reporter*, 2nd series, pp. 229–34.

Winslow, G. (1984) 'From Loyalty To Advocacy: A New Metaphor for Nursing', *The Hastings Center Report*, June, pp. 32–40.

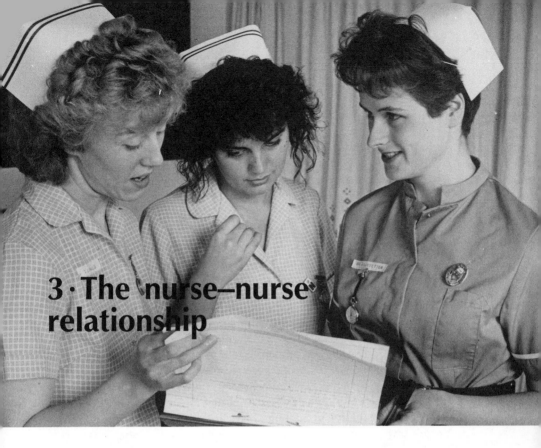

3 · The nurse–nurse relationship

Introduction

We have already noted that the Code of Conduct states, in clause 5, that each nurse shall 'work in a collaborative and cooperative manner with other health care professionals and recognise and respect their particular contributions within the health care team' (UKCC, 1984). Similarly, the ANA Code for Nurses says that nurses should 'actively promote . . . collaborative planning' (ANA, 1985, p. 16). Problems may occur, however, in working relationships between junior nurses and their seniors, or between peers. Nurse managers may face issues of a special sort. It is to these difficult areas that we now turn.

Unsafe practice

It seems clear that a basic obligation of every nurse is to avoid unsafe practice on her own account. It is difficult to think of a possible moral justification for unsafe practice. Sometimes, of course, corners are cut because of insufficient resources, but there are limits to the extent to which this should be tolerated. The Code of Conduct provides, in Clause 10, that every nurse shall:

> Have regard to the environment of care ... and make known to appropriate persons or authorities any circumstances which could place patients/clients in jeopardy or which militate against safe standards of practice.
>
> (UKCC, 1984)

The Code of Conduct further provides, in Clause 4, that in order to avoid unsafe practice a nurse should

> Acknowledge any limitations of competence and refuse in such cases to accept delegated functions without first having received instruction in regard to those functions and having been assessed as competent.
>
> (UKCC, 1984)

This may cause problems for a newly qualified nurse who is told to do something about which she is unsure, especially on a busy ward. It might appear to be the better course to avoid appearing to be a nuisance and to attempt the procedure, hoping that it will turn out all right. But there are strong ethical reasons for abiding by what the Code of Conduct says. First, applying the principle of respect for persons, if the patient knew that a nurse had little or no idea of what she was doing, he might be very unwilling to accept an intervention from that nurse. He is, in effect, being subjected to experiment without his consent. The implications of the nurse's own capacity for autonomy, moreover, are that she must accept responsibility for what she does.

If we apply a consequentialist analysis, we have to weigh up the possible consequences of complying and of refusing to comply with an order. The consequences of either course of action could be unpleasant – in the one case the anger of a senior nurse, and in the other possible damage, through incompetence, to the patient. The *likelihood* of each of these also has to be considered. To some extent, this will depend on the particular procedure involved, but it seems clear that possible damage to a patient is the worse of the two possible outcomes, and therefore should be avoided.

One of the most common dilemmas arises for nurses when confronted by unsafe practice on the part of a colleague. Issues relevant to this problem will be discussed in the context of whistle-blowing. In Chapter 1, codes were discussed and we looked at similar dilemmas for the junior nurse who sees inadequate care on the part of a nurse in a senior position.

In both these types of case, there is the problem of the authority figure. But dilemmas can also arise when unsafe practice or inadequate care is carried out by a peer, or even a junior. The problems, then, are not entirely ones of the limits of authority. On the contrary, the factors making any form of action difficult include a feeling of solidarity with a friend, or sympathy if one knows that another nurse is experiencing severe personal difficulties of some sort.

Kathleen Fenner suggests that there is an important distinction to be drawn between care that is simply less than excellent and care that is actually unsafe or harmful.

> It is one matter to observe a nurse who is rude and unfriendly, and do nothing; it is another to observe a nurse administer an incorrect medication or perform a procedure in a threatening manner, and not take appropriate action.
>
> (Fenner, 1980, p. 112)

Unless the situation is so serious that immediate action needs to be taken to protect a client, Fenner suggests that before reporting a colleague to the appropriate authorities the first step might be to share one's concern with that colleague. This may be enough to prevent a recurrence. If it is not, the matter can then be taken further. What is unacceptable, according to Fenner, is to talk about the behaviour in question with people who should not be involved in the matter.

In terms of ethical theory, Fenner's view has much to be said for it. To discuss the issue with the offending colleague shows respect for her as an autonomous agent, and this action may produce results as good, in terms of benefit to patients' interests, as reporting her immediately to seniors. The latter course of action may protect patients, but does so without showing consideration for the individual nurse, who may be alienated as a result.

It is important, however, as Fenner recognises, for channels of communication to be good, if such a system is to work. It is here that senior nurses have a major role to play in facilitating an atmosphere conducive to sharing difficulties.

Senior nurses

Hierarchies

Gena Corea, writing of American medicine, states:

> Rather than challenge the healing authority doctors established . . . nurses quietly take their place in it. They mimic doctors by setting up their own hierarchy in which the class falls lower and the skin grows darker as the jobs drop in status and power.
>
> (Corea, 1977, p. 69)

While hierarchies have their place, too rigid a reliance on authority structures can be counter-productive. A survey in the USA in 1987 found that one of the most important factors that keeps nurses in practice was being allowed to exercise nursing judgement for patient care – allowed, in other words, to exercise autonomy. The sense of being considered an important member of the health care team makes a significant contribution to the satisfaction of nurses (Katzin, 1989, p. 44). Hierarchy, without a sense of the importance of each person in the hierarchy, can fail to produce the best results for staff, and thus for patient care.

It is senior nurses who can make a difference here. Katzin quotes successful nurse managers as advocating the following approaches: keeping lines of communication open; feeling comfortable with oneself and not really being interested in status; reassuring staff that it is not a 'we/they' situation (Katzin, 1989, p. 47).

Ziel makes a related point in an article on 'the androgynous nurse manager'. Using insights from Chinese philosophy, she argues that the effective nurse manager must combine both 'yin' and 'yang'. The yang elements, associated with traditional hierarchies, include goal-directed, analytical, assertive, strategic, powerful and productive qualities. These need to be tempered however by yin: growth-oriented, creative, receptive, supportive, dedicated and collaborative qualities (Ziel, 1983).

Efficiency

It is often assumed that good management is associated with efficiency and, to a certain extent, this is true. Certainly, management that is inefficient is not good. However, as John Boatright points out, 'efficiency by the very nature of the concept cannot be a goal in itself, for it is incomplete without an answer to the question, "Efficient in doing what?"' (Boatright, 1988, p. 306).

Boatright is pointing to a very important fact about efficiency. It may be defined as taking the most effective means to chosen ends. Once this is clear, we can see that the good manager needs more than efficiency, because there is a question about whether the *right* ends are being pursued, and efficiency itself cannot set the ends. Efficiency is not an end in itself.

Boatright quotes Aristotle's view that every community is established with a view to some good (Boatright, 1988, p. 308). There may be more than one good involved, but one will be primary. In the case of the Health Service, the end in view is the health and welfare of patients, and this is reflected in the weighting given to patients' interests in the Code of Conduct. So, the good manager will be one who facilitates work towards this end. This will, of course, involve the setting-up of routines and systems, but there is always a danger that the routines and systems may come to acquire the status of ends themselves. When this happens, it is a sign that things have gone wrong. The good nurse manager will be one who provides a supportive environment in which nurses feel they have sufficient autonomy to exercise their skills in the interests of their patients.

The Code

What does this amount to in specific terms? Lois Hacker, writing in the American context, says:

> It may seem simplistic, but I believe the most basic responsibility of the nurse as an administrator or facilitator is to disseminate or distribute a copy of the Code for Nurses to each nurse employee . . . .. This may seem a rather obvious suggestion. In reality, however, at least personally, I can remember having been exposed to and instructed regarding the code only several years ago, when I was a student.
>
> (Hacker, 1978, p. 23)

Hacker is suggesting that the Code should be made a 'living' document, and further advocates that it should be incorporated in job descriptions (Hacker, 1978, p. 25).

It is important, however, for nurse managers to remember that they are themselves subject to the UKCC Code of Conduct. Clause 11, previously discussed in the context of diligence, appears to have special application to those in authority, providing that every nurse shall:

> Have regard to the workload of and the pressures on professional colleagues and subordinates and take appropriate action if these are seen to be such as to constitute abuse of the individual practitioner and/or to jeopardise safe standards of practice.
>
> (UKCC, 1984)

Again, this can be accounted for by going back to first principles. Much has been written about the obligation of practitioners to show respect for the patient as a person; less has been said about the potential abuse of practitioners themselves. Clause II of the Code of Conduct draws attention to this. Each practitioner is also a person to whom the principle of respect for persons applies. To fail to observe limits on what should be expected of individuals is to fail to treat those individuals with respect, because it is to omit to consider the world from their point of view and to make allowance for the strain they may be under.

From a consequentialist viewpoint, overloading staff may lead to disastrous results for the practitioner's health and wellbeing, and for patient care. The overstretched person, obviously, cannot give as much care as she would like to patients and will be tempted to cut corners. This may result in less than perfect and dangerous care.

There is potential for conflict here. On the one hand, the nurse manager has to see that a certain amount of work is done, with a given number of nurses to assist her. So she has a problem of allocation of resources: each must take a share of the work. There may be no way of allocating it without putting what seem to be intolerable burdens on individuals.

It is arguable, here, that the nurse manager has a special responsibility to draw attention to the inadequacy of resources, as charge nurse Pink did in relation to the lack of staffing in an elderly care ward (Guardian, 11 April 1990). While the Code of Conduct states that every nurse has this responsibility, the nurse manager may have greater access to appropriate channels.

However, the question can be asked: what are nurses supposed to do in the meantime? It is all very well saying that representations must be made to the appropriate authorities about lack of resources, but in the absence of any extra resources being allocated, how are they to continue? One answer is that they should endeavour to do the best they can under difficult circumstances. The problem is that if it is known that nurses are likely to respond in this way, the need to do anything about the shortage of resources will seem less urgent to those with the power to intervene.

Another alternative is to go on strike, an issue which raises the question of the extent to which nurses should become politically involved. This topic must now be examined.

Political involvement

The American Nurses' Association Code for Nurses, Clause 11, states that 'The nurse collaborates with members of the health professions and other citizens in promoting community and national efforts to meet the health care needs of the public' (ANA, 1985, p. 16). The interpretive statement to this clause further provides that:

> For the benefit of the individual client and the public at large, nursing's goals and commitments need adequate representation. Nurses should ensure this representation by active participation in decision-making in institutional and political arenas to assure a just distribution of health care and nursing resources.
>
> (ANA, 1985, p. 16)

But, as Sara Fry points out, this leads to some difficult choices for the nurse manager:

> The nurse manager may have to decide whether to support efforts at cost-effectiveness of health care which might decrease the quality of health care services. The nurse manager may also have to decide whether one's position on matters of professional importance is too costly in terms of potential loss of collaborative support from other health colleagues, especially the medical profession.
>
> (Fry, 1985, p. 63)

Gena Corea has described the case of Thomas Daley, a nursing director in Philadelphia, who was fired in 1974 for refusing to reprimand a nurse in accordance with a doctor's wishes (Corea, 1977, p. 66). This led to the picketing of the hospital by nurses carrying signs bearing messages such as 'Nurse Patients, Not Doctors'.

By what criteria should such conflicts be resolved? Fry suggests that the nurse manager has to decide whether a particular stance is 'too costly'. This suggests a consequentialist approach. But how are the consequences to be evaluated?

One policy that might be thought appropriate for the nurse manager is always to support the nurses against other groups of health care professionals. There are problems with this, however. First, on one view of morality, there is a close connection between morality and impartiality. To have a policy of siding always with the nursing perspective might be held to violate that. On the other hand, it might be held that it is an important part of the role of nurse manager to represent nursing interests. However, the nurse manager also has the responsibility of cooperating with the other groups of health care professionals.

How can this conflict be resolved? We have seen and shall see over and over again, that the primary responsibility of every nurse, nurse managers included, is to protect the interests of patients. So, in any conflict situation this is the criterion that must be used. And it was this criterion that led Daley to support his nurse in the case described by Corea. She writes:

> A nurse questioned a doctor's mineral-oil order for an elderly
> burns patient because she feared that the oil, in combination
> with another drug the doctor had prescribed, could cause oil
> emboli in the liver and spleen. According to Daley,
> pharmacology literature upheld the nurse's judgement.
>
> (Corea, 1977, p. 65)

Daley argued that it was the nurse's duty to question a doctor's treatment if she thought it detrimental to the patient.

The question of strike action poses particular difficulties, however. It is sometimes argued that nurses should not go on strike because to do so puts the interests of particular groups of patients at risk. On the other hand, it is argued that a strike may be the only way to draw attention to the inadequacy of resources, which is also detrimental to patients' interests. If we try to adopt the criterion of resolving conflict by looking at the patients' interests, we may find it of little help. Both striking and not striking can be defended on the grounds of patients' interests: it is a choice between protecting patient interests in the short-term and in the long-term. Different groups of patients will, of course, be involved, and this is a very difficult decision to make. The right course of action will depend on a calculation, in specific circumstances, of whether the benefit to be gained by the strike will outweigh the harm done. While a strike may be a last resort, after other channels of complaint have been used, to say that a nurses' strike can never be justified is hardly a tenable position. Such a policy encourages exploitation of nurses and provides little or no incentive to improve conditions and resources for either staff or patients (Chadwick, 1989).

The cases

Incompetence

❝ About half an hour later the old lady died ❞

The following incident occurred on a medical ward. I was helping a staff nurse with some female patients. The staff nurse was nearing retirement and maintained that she was unable to be very helpful when lifting patients or moving them about, due to a pain in her back. However, she did not inform the ward sister of this fact.

One of the patients we were looking after was a woman in her seventies, not too steady on her feet and very obese. She was frequently asking for the commode. I could see that the staff nurse was becoming increasingly impatient with her. When the old lady wanted to get back into bed we lifted her off the commode and I found myself taking most of the weight. Suddenly the staff nurse let go of the patient altogether. As she was too heavy for me to support by myself we both half fell on to the bed. By this time the patient was panicking and becoming extremely distressed, crying and wailing. The staff nurse became very angry with the patient and was very rude to her. I asked the staff nurse to help me get the patient onto the bed but she said she couldn't help me because of her back. She did give some 'assistance' by pulling the patient roughly onto the bed. In the end we managed to get her into a half sitting, half lying position on the bed. By now the old lady was hysterical. I tried to comfort her but the staff nurse just kept on being rude to her. I then left the room and found sister. I told her that the staff nurse needed some help with a patient who was very distressed. About half an hour later, the old lady died.

Commentary

In discussing this case, it is necessary to be careful to avoid the implication that the incident under consideration in some way caused or hastened the death of the patient. We do not have sufficient evidence to draw this conclusion. What we do know is that the events caused a patient considerable distress, and that the staff nurse was rude to the patient when her own back condition was largely the source of the problem.

The author of the case study implies that she thinks the correct course of action, on the part of the staff nurse, would have been to have informed the ward sister of her condition. This action, presumably, could have prevented the staff nurse from being involved in situations in which she would have to do any heavy lifting and in which her back was likely to be a handicap. It is difficult to see what reasons there could be for not doing this. Perhaps the fact that she was nearing retirement had the psychological effect of making her think that what happened at work was less important than her own needs. However, to those receiving care it is irrelevant; their needs will clearly not go away.

The junior nurse is faced, then, with a dilemma. If she follows Fenner's advice, she will ask herself whether what she is witnessing is care that is less than excellent or care that is unsafe (Fenner, 1980, p. 112). In practice, the boundaries between the two will not always be clear. The fact that this patient dies, despite our word of caution about the links of cause and effect, may influence us into thinking that this is an example of unsafe practice.

Let us assume, for the sake of argument, that it is unsafe practice – what should the junior nurse do? Fenner recommends sharing her concern with the colleague before reporting her. In this case, she has chosen to do neither of these things directly. She first tries to change her ways by setting an example – she tries to comfort the old lady, but this has no effect. She then leaves to ask the sister to help the staff nurse.

Given the position of the junior nurse in the hierarchy, this course of action possibly has the highest likelihood of achieving a good result. She has tried to act to protect the interests of the patient.

Has she violated the rights of the staff nurse? The latter may be put in a position where she is forced to disclose the condition of her back. But there is no convincing argument to the effect that she has the right to keep this private, when it is affecting her work and harming the interests of patients. Thus, in this case it appears that the junior nurse took the correct course of action, morally speaking.

Poor supervision of inexperienced nurse

❛ The staff nurse shouted 'stop!' ❜

On my first day on my first ward I was told to give an insulin injection to a patient. I was not supervised and I had never given an injection before. I did not know the patients and was just told to give the injection to 'that patient over there' by the staff nurse. I was extremely nervous, so just went up to who I thought she meant and explained to her what I was doing. I pierced the skin with the needle when the staff nurse at the other end of the ward shouted 'Stop!' Fortunately none of the insulin was injected. I apologised to the patient and then the staff nurse realised her mistake in letting me go alone to give the injection.

Commentary

We have noted that the Code of Conduct states that every nurse shall acknowledge limitations of competence and refuse to accept delegated functions without first having been assessed as competent. This case makes it clear that competence does not apply only to the ability to carry out procedures. The nurse may have been quite capable of actually administering an injection, but had no idea about the patients in the ward or to whom she ought to give the insulin.

The author nicely illustrates in this account the general point that procedures are meaningless in the absence of some understanding of the context of care, some knowledge of the patient. While this case may be atypical, mistakes of this kind are clearly more likely to occur unless there is a commitment to the care of the whole person rather than to a philosophy of administering procedures to patients stripped of their histories and personalities. It is part of the principle of respect for persons that the attempt is made to view the patient as a whole.

From the point of view of the staff nurse, we can see that article 11 of the Code of Conduct could be invoked. In its statement that every nurse shall have regard to the pressures on subordinates, it can be read as requiring sensitivity not just to excessive workloads, but also to the pressures of being new on the ward.

Retribution and reparation

❬ The student supervisor never learned that he died ❭

An improperly supervised nursing student gave 10.0 mg digitoxin (instead of 0.1 mg) to a 64-year-old man admitted to the hospital for a minor surgical procedure. Although the patient questioned the student about why he was to take so many tablets, he was reassured by the student that the doctor had ordered them. At 4 p.m., during nursing student rounds, the mistake was discovered. By that time, 8 hours had elapsed since the patient took the pills, and he had developed life-threatening arrhythmias. He was brought to the coronary care unit (CCU). A pacemaker was inserted and other supportive therapy was instituted. Nevertheless, after 8 days he died. He was aware of the error; his family was aware; the medical and nursing staff of the hospital (and the administrative staff) were aware. The patient did not want any punitive action to be brought against the student.

As a staff nurse in the CCU, I cared for this gentle person until he died. He was intelligent and alert until the end. He suffered a great deal during those 8 days. The nursing student never visited him. The student supervisor never visited and never asked the hospital for a status report; never learned that he died (unless she read it in the newspaper). The nursing supervisor was not sanctioned in any way by the hospital or by the nursing profession and indeed, was supervising another group of students the following semester on the same unit.

I wanted to have both the supervisor and the student made aware of the consequences of their error and to have some safeguards instituted to prevent a recurrence. My nursing supervisor said it was none of my business and we all make mistakes. She advised me to let the issue drop.

Commentary

This case occurred in the American context, which is generally recognised to be one in which patients are more likely to take legal action, so it is particularly significant that the patient in question did not want any action to be taken here.

What is the appropriate response of one nurse to another in such a case? Should she simply forget it, as her supervisor advises? Or is she right to feel that those whose mistake has allegedly cost a patient his life should be made to face the consequences?

Some take the view, as indicated in Chapter 2, that when one person's deliberate wrongdoing or negligence has harmed another, that retribution is deserved. In other words, the individual should be made to suffer in some way. This view is not only harsh – after all, we do all make mistakes – but seems unlikely to achieve any positive results. Of course, it may bring pleasure to those who would like to see the perpetrator suffer, but should this kind of pleasure be encouraged?

A more positive view is perhaps that the person responsible should be expected to make some sort of reparation, or amends, to the victim. It is in the light of this that the author's desire that the student nurse and/or her supervisor should visit the patient is to be understood. It was too late to save the man's life, but not too late to show regret.

What the nurse writer is specially concerned about, however, is that this should not happen in future. This represents the third view which is that the individual responsible for the mistake should be made to face the consequences in order to try to improve standards of patient care in the future. It is this that gives the nurse writer the right to speak on the case. The supervisor has told her that it is none of her business. If she had simply wanted to see people punished then that view would be understandable. However, if she is concerned that standards are threatened, when action could be taken, then arguably that is the business of every nurse.

It could be argued that the shock of realising what had happened would do as much good as any formal approach to the incident could. But what the nurse here is concerned about is that there is no evidence that those involved have any genuine realisation of what they have done.

Response to error, then, should not be concerned simply with punishment for its own sake, or be covered up out of loyalty to members of one's own profession, but it should also involve any appropriate action for maintaining and improving standards of care.

Conclusion

We have seen that relationships between nurses should be governed by the same principles that govern relationships with other people generally – that is, a respect for autonomous persons and concern for their interests. But sometimes there will be a clash between the interests of other nurses and the interests of patients. Here, because of the nature of nursing, the interests of patients must take priority.

References

American Nurses' Association (1985) *Code for Nurses with Interpretive Statements* (Kansas: ANA).

Boatright, J. R. (1988) 'Ethics and the role of the manager', *Journal of Business Ethics*, vol. 7, pp. 303–12.

Chadwick, R. F. (1989) 'Uncaring angels', *Philosophy Today*, vol. 3, p. 3.

Corea, G. (1977) *The Hidden Malpractice: How American Medicine Treats Women as Patients and Professionals* (New York: William Morrow).

Fenner, K. M. (1980) *Ethics and Law in Nursing: Professional Perspectives* (New York: Van Nostrand Reinhold).

Fry, S. T. (1985) 'The nurse manager and political involvement: individual vs. collective responsibilities', *Bioethics Reporter*, vol. 6/7, pp. 62–9.

Guardian, 'Yours sincerely, F. G. Pink', 11 April 1990.

Hacker, L. J. (1978) 'The Code for Nurses: A Nursing Administration Perspective', in American Nurses' Association, *Perspectives on the Code for Nurses*, 23–5 (Kansas: ANA).

Katzin, L. (1989) 'Great head nurses', *American Journal of Nursing*, vol. 89, pp. 43–7.

United Kingdom Central Council for Nursing, Midwifery and Health Visiting (1984) *Code of Professional Conduct for the Nurse, Midwife and Health Visitor*, 2nd ed. (London: UKCC).

Ziel, S. (1983) 'The androgynous nurse manager', *Journal of Continuing Nurse Education*, vol. 14, pp. 27–31.

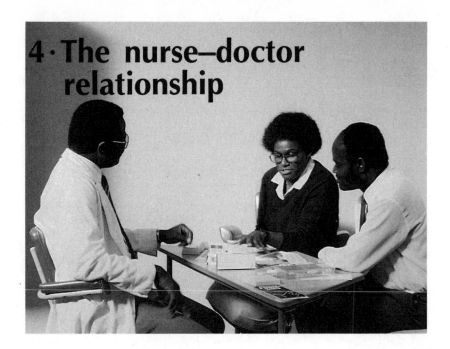

4 · The nurse–doctor relationship

Introduction

The doctor, nurse and patient constitute the fundamental triad of the health care system, and much has been written about the traditional structure and roles of the participants. Characteristically the doctor has been portrayed as 'all-knowing' and powerful; the nurse as caring, unselfish, obedient and submissive; and the patient as helpless and utterly trusting.

Currently, this situation is changing as professional barriers are being eroded and roles and structures become more flexible and less prescribed. With advances in nursing knowledge and increasing numbers of nurses following degree programmes, nurses have begun to recognise their own expertise, knowledge and their ability to make independent decisions regarding the nursing care of patients.

In addition, over the last six or seven years, the statutory body for nursing, midwifery and health visiting has placed increasing demands on individual practitioners, in terms of professional responsibility in the form of the *Code of Professional Conduct* (UKCC, 1984) and supplementary advisory documents such as *Exercising Accountability* (UKCC, 1989).

Patients are beginning to question and challenge both nursing and medical decisions made on their behalf and are expressing a right to be consulted and involved in decision-making regarding their own health and welfare. The clinical freedom of the doctor is increasingly being challenged with calls for more effective use of resources, the advent of clinical audit and the increasing public interest and political interference in the health care arena.

One result of these changes is that the professionals themselves are feeling increasingly under threat and in such conditions relationships alter.

Life is often easier when one can hide behind the responsibility of another, and there is no doubt that some nurses preferred the situation when it was acceptable to reply, 'I'm only doing what the doctor told me to do.'

On the other hand, doctors who are experts in the scientific aspects of diagnosis and treatment of disease, may well feel much more comfortable when they can distance themselves from the human and ethical dimensions of their work and assume their position of authority on the basis of superior knowledge. However, luxuries such as these are no longer possible or appropriate. To commence our examination of the nurse–doctor relationship, it is necessary to explore the concepts of power and authority.

Power

In their book *Politics of Nursing*, Kalisch and Kalisch (1980) state that the word 'power' is used continually and intuitively in everyday speech. However, when one comes to define power it is readily seen that it is an elusive concept.

 For the purposes of this discussion we can do little better than follow de Jouvenal, who defined power as the 'capacity to make others do what one wants them to do against their own desires and preferences and against their wills' (de Jouvenal, 1957, p. 32).

As already stated, the locus of power in health care has always been invested in the doctor and it is worth considering some of the sociological explanations of this situation.

Early writers, such as Durkheim and Parsons, emphasised the ethical nature of the professions, placing great importance on service to the community and specialist knowledge, suggesting that they represented the institutionalisation of altruistic values.

Sociologists, such as Hughes (1958) and Friedson (1970), challenged these approaches based on idealism and highlighted instead the benefits that follow as a result of occupational monopoly. The power dimensions of professional practice have been further developed in both Marxist and feminist accounts of the role of the professions in society and, in particular, the medical profession. (Willis, 1983; Ehrenreich and English, 1973 and 1978.)

Medical dominance has largely resulted from three strategies; subordination, limitation and exclusion (Turner, 1985, pp. 38–47). Subordination describes the ability of doctors to delegate certain activities to allied occupations thereby denying them autonomy, which is in fact the case with nursing.

Limitation involves the restriction of an occuption to either one part of the body as is the case with opticians and dentists or to a particular form of treatment such as pharmacy or physiotherapy. Frequently, doctors are involved as members of registration boards for these occupations and can, therefore, limit practice to within specific and narrow aspects of care.

Exclusion involves the denial of legitimisation by refusing registration of certain types of practitioners and examples abound in the area of alternative medicine. It is, however, interesting to note that as public interest and willingness to attempt alternative therapies grow, increasing numbers of doctors are offering wide ranges of treatments, including acupuncture, hypnosis and others.

Understanding how a profession can retain its power does not, however, explain why it should have it in the first place and this is largely to do with the nature of medical knowledge.

The acquisition of a body of specialised knowledge is one of the reasons why a profession can demand a special status within society. To retain its knowledge and the associated privilege, the profession must ensure that the knowledge cannot be rationalised or routinised and therefore subjected to external controls. An appropriate safeguard is to argue that the professional must possess the knowledge as well as being able to interpret it, and it is in the interpretation that the mystique and exclusivity lies. The interpretation of information provides a formidable barrier to external interference, as well as increasing the dependence of the client upon the professional and, hence, the professional's power is greater (Turner, 1987, p. 136).

Having considered the reasons why so much power is invested in the medical profession and the ways in which it has been able to retain it, there are two further observations to make. First, simply because one person has power it does not follow that another individual is powerless. There is not, in other words, a finite amount of power. Because one group of health professionals, namely doctors, holds power this in itself does not relegate all other health professionals to a position of being powerless.

Second, power may not be legitimate as when an armed robber wields a knife and demands 'Your money or your life', or a terrorist kidnaps an innocent bystander and holds him hostage. Although it may be legitimate for doctors to exert power and influence over the medical aspects of care, it does not follow that they should also dictate other aspects of care. When issues are of an ethical nature the doctor has no particular expertise and, therefore, it is argued should not not hold power.

Having considered some aspects of power, another important concept is that of authority.

Authority

Authority carries with it notions of legitimacy. In other words, there is the assumption that the individual exercising authority has the right to do so, as evidenced by Hobbes 'So that by authority is always understood a right of doing any act' (Hobbes, 1968, p. 218).

It follows that if someone has a right to do something, then that right ought to be respected and, thus, one ought to obey the commands or demands of a legitimate authority. When authority is viewed in such a way it can be seen that power would be a natural consequence.

However, the term authority is used in two distinct ways. For Hobbes, authority is a *de jure* concept (see glossary) as the term indicates that someone has a right to do something as for example when someone's role or the rules within an organisation places him in a position of authority.

A second sense in which the term authority is used was espoused by de Jouvenal when he stated 'What I mean by the term authority is the ability of a man to get his proposals accepted' (1957, pp. 29–31). In this sense, authority suggests the ability to influence. A common example cited in the literature is during a crisis such as a fire in a cinema when a member of the public gets everyone to file out in an orderly fashion. Being neither an off-duty firemen or the cinema manager, such a person would *exercise authority*, even though he was not *in authority* (Benn and Peters, 1959, p. 20).

This sense of authority is termed *de facto* authority (see glossary) and refers to situations when an individual in fact possesses authority even though he may not claim a right to do so.

Moving on from the different ways in which the term authority is used, Max Weber described three types of authority which depend upon the claims or bases for legitimacy (Weber, 1947, pp. 300–1).

● *Traditional authority* is legitimated by referring to old customs, as it rests 'on an established belief in the sanctity of immemorial traditions and the legitimacy of the status of those exercising authority under them' (Weber, 1947, pp. 300–1). An example of traditional authority would be that of the modern monarchy in Britain.

● *Lego-rational authority* is legitimised by an appeal to rules and laws and an example would be 'the British government [which] has authority because it was elected by a legal process and because it works within the laws of the land' (Renwick and Swinburn, 1980, p. 55).

● The third type of authority derives from the personal attributes or achievements of a particular individual. Weber called this *charismatic authority* and history has seen many such figures, such as Jesus, Napoleon or Winston Churchill.

Obviously, authority is necessary in many aspects of both public and personal life such as in employment or in living justly and fairly with one another in a community, but authority is not compatible with all areas of human activity. For example, Peters suggests that it is inappropriate in scientific and moral endeavours (Peters, 1967, p. 94). In the case of scientific theories, these are proved by experiment and observation and not by appealing to a particular individual.

Equally, morality cannot be determined by someone merely stating that one action is right over another. For philosophers, such as Immanuel Kant, there can be no moral authority, at least not in the *de jure* sense, as this would result in a loss of autonomy and a need to surrender the right to decide rationally between competing moral principles. This does not mean, however, that one cannot listen to or use guidance from those with a sound knowledge of ethical principles and theories. As Watt points out, 'there is no moral point in isolating ourselves from wise counsel' (Watt, 1982, p. 63).

Authority and power in the nurse–doctor relationship

What does this discussion of the concepts of authority and power mean for the nurse–doctor relationship?

One of the first points to make is that if authority is not legitimate, then there may be no requirement to obey. As already pointed out, doctors are rightly authorised to write medical orders and should expect to have these obeyed as for example in the prescribing of a particular drug or treatment. They do not, however, have a right to order a nurse to lie or deceive or undertake procedures which are of a dubious nature. In fact, both the *Code of Professional Conduct* and *Exercising Accountability* make it quite clear that the nurse is responsible for her own actions. The excuse of 'merely obeying orders' will not do.

Consider a situation in which a patient has been prepared for theatre and the nurse discovers that the doctor has simply presented the consent form for signing without adequately informing the patient of the procedure to be undertaken or of the possible consequences. The nurse has a duty to have 'the situation remedied' (UKCC, 1989, p. 10), and is within her rights to refuse to cooperate in the procedure.

A second and important point is that there are always limits to authority, regardless of its legitimacy. Imagine a doctor prescribing the wrong dosage of a drug and when questioned by the nurse exerting pressure on her to obey. In this instance, the nurse must withstand the pressure and refuse to act on the doctor's orders as his authority to prescribe is only legitimate if he prescribes the drug correctly, which includes the dosage.

The next issue concerns the extent of medical authority and, as already mentioned, this is limited to clinical concerns. Much of health care, however, extends beyond this sphere and encroaches on the realms of moral rather than medical decision-making. Does the nurse have to obey the doctor in such instances? Some nurses may be happy to reduce ethical concerns, such as whether to lie to patients, to the area of clinical judgement, but for many this is seen as evading the issue and shirking moral responsibility. It needs to be remembered that the nurse does not cease to be a moral agent when she goes on duty.

A challenge from the doctor may be that just as he is not an expert in ethical matters, neither is the nurse. The issue remaining however is that one's moral actions should result from deliberation and rational analysis of the principles concerned and not from merely doing as one is bid.

These conflicts cannot be resolved solely on the basis of one agent exercising authority and power over another, but instead necessitates a cooperative and collaborative approach in which the professional relationship would flourish. This would entail mutual respect and trust for the knowledge, expertise and skills that each brings to the situation.

Before going on to explore some cases which involve particular aspects of the nurse–doctor relationship it may be helpful and opportune to consider an activity which is gaining increasing interest in the nursing literature and which is particularly relevant to any discussion of professional roles and relationships, that of 'whistle-blowing'.

Whistle-blowing

Blowing the whistle refers to the act of calling to public attention abuses or dangers which jeopardise public safety and which would not otherwise be publicised. In health care, this may involve informing on the incompetent, unethical or negligent practices of colleagues, but there are powerful influences which make this much easier to discuss than to do in practice.

Bok suggests that there are three important aspects of whistle-blowing and these are dissent, accusation and breach of loyalty (Bok, 1980, pp. 2–10).

Dissent involves publicly disagreeing with authority in order to call attention to the irregularity, thereby safeguarding the public from threat. Obviously, before declaring one's dissent it is essential that the circumstances and facts surrounding the alleged abuse are accurate, as hearsay and intuition are inadequate grounds.

Deciding to inform on one's colleagues involves serious moral conflicts, one of which is breach of loyalty. Loyalty was viewed as an essential attribute of the 'good' nurse until at least the latter half of this century, as was previously mentioned in Chapter 2. Even today, being part of a health care team often involves accepting such values as not violating team loyalty.

Society generally does not hold with informing, hence the use of such labels as 'grass', 'tell-tale', 'squealer' and the like. It can be seen, therefore, that the pressure to conform to the demands of loyalty are very great and so blowing the whistle should always be used as a last resort.

Finally, one needs to consider the accusation. An accusation should identify those who are responsible rather than be couched in vague terms. It should also be made openly as anonymous accusations are unfair to the accused. As highlighted in the discussion of the nurse–nurse relationship, gossiping or making irresponsible remarks about a fellow professional are a form of injustice and can seriously damage the individual's professional reputation without offering the opportunity for the person accused to defend himself.

Before deciding to blow the whistle the individual should consider a number of questions. One is whether the benefit of 'going public' will outweigh the potential harm. A great deal of public mistrust may result which in the end may be more harmful than the original abuse. Personal harm can befall the individual who decides to complain and in many cases this has been substantial, including physical injury, loss of employment and loss of reputation.

A second point for consideration is whether publicising the problem will bring about improvements or merely ensure that in future it will be more difficult to complain. Virginia Beardshaw in her book, *Conscientious Objectors at Work* identifies a checklist of 24 points which potential whistle-blowers should consider before going public and these help to highlight just how serious a matter it is when one decides to make a public complaint (Beardshaw, 1981, pp. 99–101).

The difficulties surrounding 'whistle-blowing' do not mean that it is not possible to take any action. Nurses are bound by the *Code of Professional Conduct* to report unsafe practices and this reporting needs to be responsible. This means that written documentation should be kept of the incidents with details of who the report was made to. If no action is taken, then the report should be taken further up the organisational hierarchy until all avenues have been fully exhausted and only when this has been done should whistle-blowing be considered.

Institutions themselves should have clear guidelines for reporting, so that staff will feel supported and encouraged to share any anxieties they may have about standards of patient care. Only in this way will nurses be able to obey the moral imperative to act in the patient's interest.

The cases

Acting in the doctor's interests

❛I felt part of the whole conspiracy❜

Mr R was an 82-year-old who had had emergency abdominal surgery. During surgery, he had breathing difficulties which necessitated the insertion of a mini-tracheostomy tube. On his return to the ward, his condition was very poor and it was decided that he should not be resuscitated in the event of an arrest. Later that evening I noticed that one of the sutures anchoring the tracheostomy tube was missing and I repeatedly asked the doctor to come and replace it. Later, when attending Mr Roberts I saw that the tube was missing.

The doctor came to the ward and an X-ray revealed that the tube was lying in the patient's right bronchus. The medical team decided to perform a bronchoscopy, but to do so needed consent. They called the man's son and told him a further investigation was essential and naturally he gave his consent.

During the procedure Mr Roberts arrested and was resuscitated after which he was transferred to the intensive care unit. After 24 hours he was returned to the ward and died a few hours later.

This patient was kept alive to save the houseman and his son was totally unaware of the risks or exactly why his father had to go to theatre. I knew what was happening, but I felt powerless to say anything. When Mr Roberts died I was unable to comfort his son as I felt part of the whole conspiracy.

Commentary

One of the reasons that this nurse is experiencing moral distress in relation to this man's treatment is that she believes that the patient has been deliberately kept alive to avoid the necessity of a coroner's inquest which would have been the case had he died within 24 hours of surgery. No doubt had this event occurred the houseman would have had to answer some difficult questions as to why he had not secured the tube and the whole truth would have had to be told to the relatives.

Another of her concerns is that the decisions to resuscitate the patient and to transfer him to the intensive care unit were not taken because they were in the patient's best interests, but because they were in the doctor's.

She seems to have good reasons for making this assumption as, when first admitted, the decision was taken that active resuscitation was not appropriate should a cardiac arrest occur. Only after removal of the missing tube was the decision reversed and added to by transferring the patient to the intensive care unit where he was kept alive for the required time before being returned to the ward and allowed to die. Such treatment is clearly a means of achieving the doctor's goal rather than of treating Mr Roberts correctly.

A second aspect of the nurse's unease is her knowledge that the relatives had been deliberately misled as to the reasons behind the further intervention and that they were not informed of the risks that this entailed.

As a junior member of the caring team, the nurse feels unable to complain either internally or to the relatives by informing them of the truth. Although one can understand the awesomeness of standing up to medical authority, one also needs to ask whether such silence is in fact justifiable.

Some nurses may wish to argue that having reported to the doctor that the tube was loose, the nurse had discharged her obligations and that from there on the decisions were the doctors and, thus, no concern of hers.

Others, however, may suggest that such an approach would qualify as a classic example of the 'clean hand syndrome' and, as such, would not relieve the nurse of her moral responsibilities to either the patient or his relatives.

This view of morality suggests that one has obligations to act even when one merely observes morally culpable actions on the part of others. The excuse that one played no direct part in the action, but was only a bystander, is not acceptable. Consider the man on duty outside the gas chamber in a Nazi concentration camp: he could claim that he neither turned on the gas nor chose who was to enter, but would we accept such arguments in his defence?

It is often comfortable to believe that one is powerless in the face of difficult situations as this means that one can ignore them. But nurses must be aware of reducing ethical decisions to either clinical or medical ones and of claiming to be powerless in an attempt to avoid shouldering one's moral responsibilities.

Perhaps the very least that could have been done in this case was for the nurse to have expressed her disagreement with the way in which the patient's care was handled. The relatives could have been prompted, if not encouraged, to ask more searching questions about why more 'investigations' were required.

Nurses often fail to recognise that because they form the interface between patients, their relatives and doctors, they are in fact very powerful. By educating patients and their families to ask pertinent questions, this power could be effectively transferred to the patient enabling him or his relatives to obtain relevant information.

Accidents and unfortunate incidents do and will continue to happen in health care as in other walks of life. However, what is most disturbing in this incident is the covert manner in which things have been handled, giving substance to the old joke about doctors burying their mistakes.

An argument that might be put forward is that following the patient's death, no-one's interests would be served by either appraising the relatives of the facts or making a formal complaint about the medical treatment. Anyone putting forward such a justification, however, would need to affirm that they would be equally happy if a disaster such as Lockerbie were dealt with in a similar manner.

The aim of establishing an enquiry is to determine the cause of such public tragedies and to ensure, as far as possible, that such errors do not occur in the future by raising the issues to the level of public awareness.

Nurses also have a duty to society and so their concerns must not only rest with their individual patients but should encompass safe-guarding the interests of future patients.

Within society it is generally accepted that individuals are seen to be accountable for their actions, and this should apply as equally to medical practitioners as it does to the employees of Pan American or any other airline. For those who wish to say that the analogies are false, as the tragedy referred to involved hundreds of dead and injured, then it is worth pointing out that if we consider the numbers of people admitted to our hospitals each year, the potential for human misery and disaster is enormous.

It is interesting to ponder how, if this man's son discovered the truth, he would have judged the nurse's complicity in the affair, for the nurse clearly feels that she has played a part in the deception.

If someone merely observes a crime then obviously they are not guilty of it. If later they are involved in covering up the crime, then they are liable to be accused of being an accessory. Certainly the nurse did not word the request for consent, nor did she lie to relatives, but she knowingly omitted to inform them! The nurse presumably did not play an active part in the decision-making but again she omitted to complain on the patient's behalf.

What is at issue is whether or not omissions are morally as culpable as actions. Though philosophical opinions differ on this subject, certainly within the realms of health care one must ask whether or not the omission is intentional? If it is, then it seems logical to assert that as such it must count, at least ethically, as a responsible action as an alternative course is always available.

It appears then that just as the doctors safe-guarded their own interests by omitting to admit to their errors, so the nurse chose the easy option and omitted to act in the interests of the patient, his relatives or future patients.

As we have already identified, it is not easy to criticise openly those who are perceived as powerful, but ethical behaviour is not always easy, especially for those with a duty to the general public. It is perhaps worth remembering those civil servants such as Clive Pontin who 'blew the whistle' on the government rather than be part of the conspiracy to conceal information. Equally, it is worth recalling that in the Pontin case, the jury refused to find him guilty despite being directed to do so by the judge. This clearly demonstrates where public opinion lies with regard to conspiracy and the disclosure of information.

Nurses must ask themselves whether or not they are contributing to the unauthorised power of medical practitioners by complying with their decisions and thus appearing to condone such behaviour.

Orders to lie

❛I believed she had a right to the truth❜

Sarah was 40 years of age, she had an inoperable brain tumour and had less than a year to live. Her husband had been informed and requested that his wife not be told of the medical findings.

The doctors agreed with these wishes and the nursing staff were to say nothing. Doctors, nurses, the family, even the ward domestic knew of her situation, but no-one informed the woman herself.

Nursing her was impossible, especially as she repeatedly asked 'What's wrong with me', or 'Surely they must have some results now'. I, like all the other nurses had as little contact with this patient as possible and when I had to face her I was brisk, cheerful and practical. I avoided contact because as a nurse it just isn't possible to say nothing and I disliked and felt guilty about lying. I was also afraid that I would let something slip as I was never sure what exactly she had been told by the doctors or her family at any time. I believed she had a right to the truth about her own life.

Commentary

What is so special about the nurse in this case, for after all the doctors are also lying to the patient? The doctors chose to lie, be it right or wrong, and they did so willingly. Not so the nurse as she was ordered to lie.

Second, doctors, relatives and other health professionals spend significantly less time with patients than nurses do so that it is the nurse who stands in the firing line of the very difficult questions that patients naturally ask. This particular nurse correctly identifies that in such situations it is not possible to say 'nothing'. Instead, the nurse either lies, tells the truth or communicates with the patient in such a way that trust and confidence are lost.

Frequently, relatives request that unpleasant news be kept from their loved ones, but often this is from a misguided sense of protection or from a desire to spare their own sensitivity. In no other situation would a relative have the right to dictate what information may or may not be passed on to the patient, providing the patient was judged to be competent.

Doctors also commonly demand that nurses withhold the truth from terminally ill patients, using the argument that patients would not be able to cope with the information. In the USA, it is the rule that patients are told their diagnosis and there is very little evidence that patients cannot cope with such news.

A recent survey of general practitioners and their patients indicated that 80 per cent of family doctors would lie to dying patients and yet 94 per cent of the patients questioned wanted to be told if they were dying. One of the commonest reasons given for this deceit was that they just did not know how to break the bad news. Forty per cent of doctors questioned admitted that what they most wanted was for people to be less demanding (*Independent*, March, 1990).

The end result of such deception is a pathetic charade of patient care, with the patient eventually mistrusting not only the doctors and nurses involved, but also their family and friends at a time when they need to feel supported.

In situations such as these, the doctor is treating the nurse as an instrument or object, disregarding not only her own moral views and beliefs about the rightness or wrongness of her own actions, but also the professional contributions that she can legitimately make to patient care. The nurse often has considerable knowledge of the patient as a person, of his beliefs and values, integrity and human needs which can inform and improve the quality of care and treatment that is provided.

Situations which deny this valuable input militate against the nurse acting in the patient's interests and frequently lead to poor standards of care.

Conclusion

One of the major issues in the nurse–doctor relationship is who shall be the moral agent? Many nurses are no longer willing to follow blindly the doctor's orders and in the case of moral demands she may well be right in resisting. As Veatch points out, the doctor:

> must be able to distinguish technical questions of medicine,
> which are more appropriately his (her) own area of competence,
> from value dimensions, for which he (she) may or may not have
> special competence.
>
> (Veatch, 1978, p. 874)

In questions of morality, patients, nurses, doctors and other health care professionals may all make valid and important contributions and, therefore, decisions of this nature should not be made in isolation by any one member of the team. Indeed, research in the USA has shown that one of the main contributing factors to nurse burn-out is moral distress, and the more that nurses compromise their integrity, the more burned-out they become (Cameron, 1986, pp. 42B–42E).

If health care is a team venture, then each member of the team must be willing to reflect on the moral dimensions of their work and discuss openly how such issues are to be resolved.

Nurses must be more willing to make explicit their role as moral agents and doctors must be willing to listen to them. Collaboration and cooperation rather than conflict would best serve the patient's interest.

References

Beardshaw, V. (1981) *Conscientious Objectors at Work* (London: Social Audit).

Benn, S. I. and Peters, R. S. (1959) *Social Principles and the Democratic State* (London: George Allen & Unwin).

Bok, S. (1980) 'Whistleblowing and Professional Responsibility', *New York University Education Quarterly*, vol. 10.

Cameron, M. (1986) 'The Moral and Ethical Component of Nurse-Burnout', *Nursing Management*, vol. 17, no. 4, 42B–42E.

Ehrenreich, B. and English, D. (1973) *Witches, Midwives and Nurses. A History of Women Healers* (New York: Feminist Press).

Ehrenreich, B. and English, D. (1978) *For Her Own Good: A Hundred and Fifty Years of the Experts Advice to Women* (New York: Anchor Press).

Friedson, E. (1970) *Profession of Medicine: A Study of the Sociology of Applied Knowledge* (New York: Harper and Row).

Hughes, E. C. (1958) *Men and Their Work* (Glencoe: Free Press).

Hobbes, T. (1968) *Leviathan*, C. B. Macpherson (ed.) (Harmondsworth: Penguin).

Independent, 5th March 1990.

de Jouvenal, B. (1957) *Sovereignty*, J. F. Hutchinson (transl.) (Chicago: Chicago University Press).

Kalisch, B. J. and Kalisch, P. A. (1980) *Politics of Nursing* (Philadelphia: J. B. Lippincott).

Peters, R. S. (1967) 'Authority', in A. Quinton (ed.), *Political Philosophy* (London: Oxford University Press).

Renwick, A. and Swinburn, I. (1980) *Basic Political Concepts* (London: Hutchinson).

Turner, B. S. (1985) 'Knowledge, Skill and Occupational Strategies: The Professionalisation of Paramedical Groups', *Community Health Studies*, vol. 9. pp. 38–47.

Turner, B. S. (1987) *Medical Power and Social Knowledge*, London: Sage Publications). pp. 38–47.

United Kingdom Central Council for Nurses, Midwives and Health Visitors (1984) *Code of Professional Conduct*, 2nd ed. (London: UKCC).

United Kingdom Central Council for Nurses, Midwives and Health Visitors (1989) *Exercising Accountability* (London: UKCC).

Veatch, R. M. (1978) 'Medical Ethics Education', in W. T. Reich (ed.), *Encyclopaedia of Bio-ethics* (New York: The Free Press).

Watt, E. D. (1982) *Authority* (London: Croom Helm).

Weber, M. (1947) *Theory of Social and Economic Organisation*, A. M. Henderson and T. Parsons (transl.), (London: Hodge).

Willis, E. (1983) *Medical dominance, division of labour in Autralian health care* (Sydney: Allen and Unwin).

Part II

5 · Nursing adults

Introduction

Bandman and Bandman define adulthood as the period between 20 and 65 years of age, dividing this rather lengthy period of time into two phases; early adulthood (20 to 35 years of age) and middle age (35 to 65 years of age). They admit, however, that these figures are arbitrary (Bandman and Bandman, 1985, p. 186). In English law, a young person officially 'comes of age' at 18 years, so for the purposes of this discussion it will be assumed that this is when adulthood starts.

What does it mean to become an adult? Chambers' Dictionary defines 'adult' as 'grown-up' or 'mature', where 'mature' means fully developed physically, mentally and emotionally. Clearly, some people mature much earlier than others. As far as the law is concerned, however, some age has to be set at which individuals can be held liable under contracts, for example. Any boundary set will not be perfect, and in various spheres the law has taken the view that people younger than 18 years of age may be mature enough to take important decisions on their own account, as we shall see in Chapter 7.

In taking the start of adulthood to be 18 years of age, then, we are not suggesting that everyone at that age suddenly becomes mature. It is a convenient dividing line, but no more than that.

What of 65 years of age being stated as the end of adulthood? What are the implications of this? There is a view that 65 marks the beginning of old age, and the problems that arise from this will be discussed in Chapter 11.

Adult patients, who are presumed to be in full possession of their faculties, provide the central case for health care. Problems about, for example, informed consent arise in their purest form with regard to such patients.

Bandman and Bandman's suggested division of the group into two phases is important, however, for two reasons. First, it is likely that there will be a difference in the kinds of health care problems that arise for the two groups. Second, there are different generations involved. Each will be influenced in their values by their own particular experiences. Bandman and Bandman themselves point out that their 20–35-year-old group consists of people born into the nuclear age who are perhaps more likely to challenge the existing order (Bandman and Bandman, 1985, p. 186). Such influences are important for the nurse trying to take the values of her patients into account.

Autonomy

The central concept in thinking about nursing the adult is autonomy. The principle of autonomy is, of course, important in relation to other groups of patients, but in the case of adults in particular it is central, because it is in adulthood, above all, that people are thought to enjoy their fullest capacity for autonomy. Mature people, at the peak of their development, are in the best position to make genuinely autonomous choices, and because they have this capacity, the principle of autonomy tells us to respect those choices (Gillon, 1985, p. 117).

In the case of children, it is thought justifiable in many, if not all, cases to be paternalistic, on the grounds that they are less likely to choose what is best for themselves. With adults however, there is a presumption that, on the whole, they do know what is in their own best interests: that respecting their autonomy and promoting their welfare coincide. If we try to interfere with decisions that are very personal to the individual, we may make terrible, though well-meaning, mistakes. As John Stuart Mill wrote in his essay *On Liberty*:

> the strongest of all the arguments against the interference of the public with purely personal conduct, is that when it does interfere, the odds are that it interferes wrongly, and in the wrong place.
>
> (Mill, 1859, p. 102)

Informed consent

Arguments about autonomy are related to the issue of informed consent, which has been described as *the* ethical issue in medicine today (Faulder, 1985, p. 2).

> Informed consent has been defined as the patient's right to know, before agreeing to a procedure, what the procedure entails – the hazards, the possible complications, and expected results of the treatment. The patient must understand any reasonable alternatives to the proposed procedure, including, in most cases, the results that can be predicted from non-treatment.
>
> (Holder and Lewis, 1981, p. 1)

The conveying of information, however, is only one element in informed consent. The other is ensuring that a genuine consent can be given. In order for consent to be genuine, it is necessary that the patient has all the relevant information as well as being in agreement without any undue pressure or influence. If the agreement is not truly voluntary then what we have is merely assent, not consent.

The link between informed consent and autonomy is that, since mature adults are presumed to have a capacity for autonomy, there is, as Raanon Gillon points out, a moral requirement to show respect for this autonomy, and '[p]art of what such respect for autonomy implies, in practical terms, is not interfering with people without their consent – not imposing interference on people' (Gillon, 1985, p. 117). But, as Gillon recognises, and as has been suggested above, there are also reasons why informed consent might be supported on utilitarian grounds. It promotes welfare to allow people to make their own decisions, and certainly few things are likely to upset someone more than finding out, after an event which has turned out badly, that they were denied crucial information which might have made a difference to their decision.

It is advisable, however, to consider the possible arguments against the importance of informed consent, to see if they provide any justification for keeping a patient in ignorance.

First, some people argue that informed consent is a myth; that no patient could ever give genuine informed consent, because the nature of the relationship between the patient and health care professional is such that the patient can never have the same degree of understanding of relevant information.

To counter this problem, it has been suggested that the very word 'patient' should be avoided, because it suggests passive acceptance. Rather, we should speak in terms of 'client' with its implications that the person receiving care is an autonomous chooser (cf. Muyskens, 1982, p. 128). It is not clear, however, how great an impact a mere verbal change can have on the realities of relationships in health care. For there is a further argument that illness in itself diminishes the capacity for autonomy (Pellegrino, 1979). Even mature adults may be less capable of making genuinely informed, rational decisions when they are ill, and may in fact welcome others who are willing to relieve them of the burden of decision-making.

While it is true that people may be hindered in their decision-making by illness, this also applies to many sorts of pressure in life, such as stress at work, or personal unhappiness. It is unjustifiable to assume that people who are ill, any more than people who are unhappy, suddenly become incapable of autonomous choice. Some forms of mental illness are thought to render their sufferers incompetent to make choices, but the presumption should be that persons are competent until proven otherwise. The adults under discussion at present are not persons suffering from a mental illness or from a mental handicap. It is, of course, open to people to use their capacity for choice to ask someone else, such as a health care professional, what they recommend, but there is no justification for making that choice for them.

A further argument against informed consent suggests that it is not always in the best interests of the patient to be fully informed. Telling people of all the risks of a particular treatment can do actual harm. To dwell on unpleasant possibilities can make their realisation more likely – for example, if patients are told of possible side-effects they may begin to imagine that they have them.

A related argument was put forward in the Sidaway case, where a woman undergoing an operation was not warned of the 1 in a 100 risk of damage, which occurred, to her spinal cord. In the Court of Appeal, Sir John Donaldson, Master of the Rolls, said that too much information might hinder rather than help the patient in making a rational choice (*Guardian*, 1 March 1984). When the case reached the House of Lords, however, Lord Scarman expressed regret at the lack in English law of a doctrine of informed consent (*Guardian*, 22 February 1985). The test used in this case was the Bolam principle, which holds that a doctor is not being negligent if current medical opinion or practice is followed. This, in effect, gives the doctor authority to decide how much patients should be told. In his support for a doctrine of informed consent, however, Lord Scarman said that doctors should provide advice to enable a patient to make up her own mind 'unless the information would be detrimental to the patient's mental health or general health'.

This criterion, however, being vague, still seems to leave the ultimate decision-making power to doctors. Robert Veatch has prophesied that in the 1990s, as the implications of the autonomy model of health care are followed to their logical conclusion:

> it will no longer make sense for physicians to write prescriptions. The model will be one of physicians informing patients of treatment alternatives and patients deciding whether a particular intervention is appropriate, given the value judgments involved.
>
> (Veatch, 1990, p. 3)

If we believe in autonomy, then, the decision-making power must rest with the patient. According to Nora Bell there are only two exceptions to this: emergencies and situations in which the patient has specifically relinquished the right to know (Bell, 1981, p. 1171).

What are the obligations of nurses with regard to informed consent? Nurses are frequently assigned the task of taking to patients the standard hospital consent forms for operations. But, as Holder and Lewis suggest, 'informed consent is quite a different thing from the consent form' (Holder and Lewis, 1981, p. 2). They go further:

> Ethically . . . it is obvious that if a nurse knows that a patient has no idea of the nature or consequences of what is about to happen, she is obliged to take action.
>
> (Holder and Lewis, 1981, p. 2)

In their opinion, however, this does not necessarily mean taking it upon herself to inform the patient:

> The nurse's duty is to notify the physician of the patient's lack of comprehension, or, alternatively, to make the problem known

to the nursing administrator who has the authority to deal with the matter.

(Holder and Lewis, 1981, p. 8)

Is this sufficient? What if it is quite clear that the physician has no intention of informing the patient, and the nursing administrator has a policy of supporting the medical staff at all costs?

Nora Bell has argued that, in such a case, the nurse has a duty to seek to provide the patient with the information required. In discussing the Tuma case, in which a nurse discussed alternative therapies with her patient and was subsequently charged with interfering with the physician–patient relationship, Bell points out the inappropriateness of seeing that case in terms of a wrong done to the physician. As she points out, the moral considerations underlying the principle of informed consent apply equally to the nurse, and 'patients' rights should not fall before disputes over professional boundaries' (Bell, 1981, p. 1172). While the first resort is to ask the physician to provide information, the last resort is to provide it herself.

It is important to recognise that this issue applies not only to consent to treatment but also to voluntary participation in experimental programmes and to randomised clinical trials (cf. Faulder, 1985).

Justice

In health care, questions about distribution arise. These concern questions about the distribution of scarce resources, such as dialysis machines, as well as factors, such as nursing time. When there are questions about distribution, there are issues of justice.

Justice is an example of an 'essentially contested concept' (cf. Gallie, 1956) in that there are several different interpretations of justice, which are in constant and irresolvable conflict.

In this discussion, we shall limit ourselves to two conceptions of justice, which have special relevance to the issues involved when nursing adults.

Justice and equality

Many people consider that justice has some necessary connection with equality. There is a presumption that people should be treated equally, unless there is a difference between them that is relevant to the treatment in question. For example, in distributing food, there is a relevant difference between a two-year old child and a grown man that justifies us in departing from a principle of equal shares and giving larger portions to the man.

In fact, it might be argued that, if we interpret 'justice as equality' correctly, the above example does not represent a departure from the principle. The principle of equality does not tell us to treat people in exactly the same way, but to give equal consideration to equal interests, or to equal needs. In the food example, one person's needs are greater than the other's, but the needs of both are satisfied. So they have, in a sense, been treated equally in that their needs have been given equal consideration.

Problems arise when the needs of some people are given less weight than those of others for reasons that are irrelevant. In other chapters, we shall be exploring this phenomenon with regard to groups of patients other than adults. In this chapter, however, the point in question is how some adults may be treated worse than others, or discriminated against, because of irrelevant factors.

The main issues here concern sexism and racism. Race and sex differences may be relevant in some therapeutic contexts. For example, they can affect the kinds of health care problems from which a patient is likely to suffer. Cultural differences may be relevant in determining how patients should be treated: some interventions may be unacceptable to people with certain belief systems. The Code of Conduct (clause 6) provides that every nurse shall 'take account of the customs, values and spiritual beliefs of patients/clients' (UKCC, 1984). But, if certain races receive worse treatment on the grounds of racial differences alone, or if women are taken less seriously than men because, for example, they are stereotyped as particularly susceptible to 'imaginary' pains, then this is discrimination on the basis of an irrelevant difference and therefore unjust.

The American Code for Nurses is more explicit on discrimination than is the UKCC, saying:

> The need for health care is universal, transcending all national, ethnic, racial, religious, cultural, political, educational, economic, developmental, personality, role and sexual differences. Nursing care is delivered without prejudicial behaviour.
>
> (ANA, 1985, p. 3)

The UKCC Code of Conduct perhaps does not need to be so explicit. Promoting the interests of patients would be incompatible with prejudice.

It is not only patients who are at risk of racism and sexism. Nurses themselves may have to deal with sexist or racist prejudice. In particular, nursing is still predominantly a female occupation and nursing has to some extent been seen as a feminist issue (Hull, 1982; Muff, 1988).

Justice and desert

A rival way of interpreting justice is in terms of desert. Justice, it might be said, is a matter of 'getting one's just deserts'.

There are two senses in which it could be argued that not all patients are equally deserving. First, some people's ill health may be due to some feature of their lifestyle that they could have avoided – smoking, drinking heavily or sexual promiscuity, for example. Do such individuals deserve the same level of care as the fitness conscious person who 'out of the blue' is struck down by a tragic disease?

Whatever we might think of the connection between justice and 'just desert', to operate a health service on the basis of such criteria would be completely impracticable. If, for example, there is a statistically greater risk of serious injury for car drivers than for pedestrians, does it follow that pedestrians should take priority in health care? To implement such a policy would not be politically feasible. Almost everyone, in fact, takes some avoidable risks with their health, so to discriminate on the basis of 'just desert' would not be possible.

There is also a deeper objection to the 'desert' argument. The desert model of justice rests on the assumption that, as autonomous persons, we are all responsible for the choices we make. But, however much we might support autonomy as an ideal, it is essential to recognise that as a matter of fact people's choices are frequently subject to the limitations of the circumstances in which they live. It is easier for those who are well off to select healthy foods and take exercise; more difficult to give up smoking if you have few other pleasures in life.

In this sense, then, the desert model of health care is unsatisfactory. The basis of the claim to health care is that people are ill. As Bernard Williams has pointed out, '[l]eaving aside preventive medicine, the proper ground of distribution of medical care is ill health' (Williams, 1969, p. 163).

The manipulative patient

The second argument that not all people are equally deserving of justice relates to people whose conduct as patients makes them difficult. This may be because they are very demanding, noncompliant, or simply because there is a personality clash between them and their carers.

Mary Ellen McMorrow describes the behaviour of a manipulative patient who attempts to control the nursing staff through verbal abuse and attention-getting stunts (McMorrow, 1981). She asks what a nurse can do when faced with such behaviour. In cases like this, she suggests, the manipulators are really afraid of confronting their own feelings. One important response, then, is to provide the setting in which the patient can express those feelings. But, it also has to be made clear just how far they can go.

> The nurse can only help the manipulator by setting firm and clearly defined behaviour. Consistency is essential. The nursing staff must be united, since the manipulative person will play one staff member against the other.

She also stresses the importance of taking the time to gain control of the situation.

> I have found the best thing to do is to take a mini-vacation. Go for coffee. Get control of your emotions and try to determine why he is manipulating you . . .. Then, you can go back to your patient and respond to him rather than be controlled by the emotions he arouses in you.
>
> (McMorrow, 1981, p. 1190)

This is presented as good practical advice, but it also has the support of moral argument. McMorrow argues that if nurses allow themselves to be manipulated, they will not be able to meet the needs of such patients or of other patients, as they will receive care from frustrated and angry nurses. Manipulative patients must be dealt with, but the temptation, as McMorrow all too clearly describes, is to avoid them and ignore them for as long as possible. In discussing her particular case study, she says 'the nurses on the unit that usually took the open heart cases threatened to quit en masse if Gary came to their unit' (McMorrow, 1981, p. 1188).

Although it may be understandable, to respond in this way is to fail to recognise that manipulative patients, like other adults who are ill, have health care needs, and these, not 'desert', are the grounds for care.

Sexuality

To discriminate against a patient on the grounds of sexual orientation is as unjustifiable as discrimination on the grounds of race or sex, but that is not the primary area of interest under this heading. What is of concern is the difficulty that carers may have in responding to or dealing with the sexuality of their patients.

In some contexts, talk about morality is assumed to be concerned with sex. Professional ethics, to some people, might appear to be about the wrongness of sexual relationships between professional and client. The range of topics covered in this volume shows that morality, and Ethics, have a much wider area of concern. However, ethical dilemmas do arise if patients show sexual interest in a nurse, whether this is welcomed or not.

This is not, of course, a problem that arises only in relation to adults, but it is as likely to occur here as anywhere.

The issues surrounding the 'seductive' patient are discussed by Jane Assey and Joan Moore Herbert (Assey and Herbert, 1983). They point out that, in the period of convalescence, many patients feel anxious to reassess and reassert their sexuality. This is so even if their particular illness represents no particular threat to their sexuality. Illness undermines people's self-image, and hospitalised patients, depersonalised as they may be, naturally want to feel attractive and valued in this area as in others. Nurses may present a convenient target, and may be confronted by provocative words or gestures. As in the case of the manipulative patient, Assey and Herbert suggest that the nurse should examine the motives behind the behaviour, in order to meet the patient's real needs, and they give practical guidance on how this can be done, with the following aim in mind: 'The goals . . . are to stop the behaviour and to create an atmosphere in which the patient and the nurse can talk about the meaning of the behaviour' (Assey and Herbert, 1983, p. 532).

The cases

The placebo and informed consent

❛I believe it to be probably classed as an assault❜

When I was working on a surgical ward a patient was admitted with back pain. His medical notes revealed that he had a history of 'mysterious' disorders. For example, a laminectomy scar had been picked open and the sutures torn, witnessed by another patient. He was also found to hide thermometers in his bedclothes to warm them, and to hide tablets that were supposed to be taken.

After repeated requests for strong analgesia, the senior house-man decided, along with the staff nurse, to administer water as a placebo. The patient was informed that the drug was his usual medication. The patient suffered no more ill-effects until his next drugs were due in four hours' time.

This was a decision made by a senior houseman and a senior staff nurse. I was unaware if this was against the law or not. Now, I believe it to be probably classed an an assault. I refrained from interfering and had nothing to do with it. I was not consulted or asked to participate and hence considered myself removed from the act.

Commentary
This case raises issues both about informed consent and about how to deal with a manipulative patient.

Was it justifiable for the houseman and staff nurse to decide to administer water as a placebo? It is arguable that, since it appeared to work, the end justified the means. The patient, after all, did not complain of pain after receiving the water.

We cannot infer from this that he was not genuinely experiencing any pain earlier. The fact that placebos can relieve symptoms has been demonstrated. They can even produce side-effects (Collier, 1989, p. 23). The part played by the mind in healing is not well understood but is known to be considerable.

So, let us assume that the patient was genuinely feeling pain, which the administration of the placebo relieved. Does that justify the action taken, on consequentialist grounds?

It has been argued that, with regard to competent adults, the principle of informed consent should be followed. There are good grounds for this both in the notion of respect for autonomy and in utilitarianism. In this case, however, the patient has not been allowed to give informed consent. He has, in fact, been deliberately lied to, and told that he was receiving his normal medication.

The most persuasive argument against informed consent is that, in a given case, the patient is thought unlikely to choose in accordance with his best interests. In fact, that argument has been rejected here on the grounds that, when competent adults are involved, there is a presumption that they are the best judges of what is in their own interests. In the situation described above, however, it seems unlikely that the action was taken even in the *belief* that it was in the best interests of the patient. The clear implication is that it was done because the patient was regarded as manipulative, and was not believed.

People who 'cry wolf', as we know, take risks. The patient described in the article by Mary Ellen McMorrow simulated several heart attacks, to gain the nurses' attention, before dying of a real one (McMorrow, 1981). While it may be understandable, it is not justifiable to assume that there is nothing wrong with a manipulative patient and his needs should be carefully assessed at all times.

McMorrow has shown that, apart from any physical symptoms they may have, such patients have needs which are motivating their behaviour. If the patient in this case is going to such unusual lengths to attract attention, then clearly he has needs that are not being met. Anyone who has the interests of the patient at heart needs to find out what these needs are.

The author of the case study, however, feels that it is not her responsibility, as she has not participated in the act. However, the Code of Conduct points out that every nurse is responsible for both acts and omissions (UKCC, 1984), and it is arguable that the nurse, in this case, had it in her power to do something by way of protest against an unjustifiable act.

Sexuality

❛He overruled the nursing staff❜

I was nursing a patient with carcinoma of the bladder. The patient was not informed of the full effects of the operation he was to undergo. He was going to have a cystectomy and formation of the ileal conduit, as a result of which he would be impotent. The patient was relatively young, and his wife was only 40 years old. I wanted to discuss this with the patient as part of his care and wanted the medical staff to discuss the possibility of a silicone rod implant. I asked the charge nurse if this was possible and he said 'no', the consultant did not believe in telling patients the full effects as they would change their minds.

The charge nurse did not believe this was morally right: he agreed with me and the rest of the staff. The charge nurse had had numerous discussions with the consultant, but he was adamant in his belief and overruled the nursing staff.

Commentary

Issues of both informed consent and sexuality arise in this case.

First, is it justifiable to withhold such information from the patient? According to the doctrine of informed consent, of course, it is not. We have seen that in the Sidaway case a considerable body of opinion thought it acceptable to withhold details about the risks of 1 in 100, though even this view is controversial. However, in the above case, there is no suggestion that there is only a small risk of impotence.

The consultant in question withheld relevant information from his patients on the grounds that, with this knowledge, they might change their minds about the operation. The most favourable interpretation that can be put upon this is that he is acting in accordance with what he believes to be in the best interests of the patient. As J. S. Mill pointed out, over a century ago, such paternalism may well be misguided.

The patient is being denied the opportunity to make a decision about the future of his own life (for him, physical survival may not take priority over other things of value, such as his masculinity). In addition, as he does not have all the facts, he has not been given the opportunity to talk it over with his wife before the operation to give them both time to adjust. As things are, they will suffer a rude awakening after the event.

As indicated above, a person's sexuality may be so important to them that they desperately need reassurance about it when recuperating from illness. It is hardly justifiable to take away a person's ability to perform sexually without warning them of this.

What should the nurse, in this case, do? She has taken the problem to her head nurse. If persons in authority have discussed it with the consultant to no avail, and patients' interests are seen to be damaged, it is arguable that this is an example of a case when it would be justifiable for the nurse to have the discussion, to which she thinks he is entitled, with the patient.

Informed consent

❛ The doctor spoke to her as if she were a 10-year-old ❜

An 18-year-old girl had a biopsy of a growth on her clavicle. She was very withdrawn, and this was not helped by the fact that all the other patients in the ward were over 60 years of age. The doctors kept her and her family waiting for days. All the nursing staff, including myself, knew that the growth was malignant and that secondaries were very probable. One morning she was crying so I sat with her. She was quite depressed; she felt forgotten by the doctors who were just putting off telling her. When, later in the day, she was told, the doctor spoke to her as if she were a 10-year-old. The way she was told made her distrusting and confused about the medical staff. She was not told anything specific about the treatment the doctor called X-ray treatment – even though she was to have chemotherapy, nothing was explained about this or about how she might help herself. When I spoke to her she was grasping for any shreds of information I might give her. We talked about attitudes to illness, wanting to recover, and how the chemotherapy would make her ill but can be very successful.

Commentary

This case illustrates that in some cases the reason behind withholding information from a patient is self-protection on the part of the staff, rather than the best interests of the patient. Gail Young has described how doctors employ defence mechanisms to distance themselves from patients and, in this case, speaking to the young woman as if she were a 10-year-old serves this purpose (Young, 1981). There are also other issues involved, such as truth-telling, which has been discussed elsewhere. There has been a delay in passing on bad news.

The reluctance to pass on unpleasant information, however, has resulted in a failure to give the full facts to the patient and her family. Therefore, there are questions about whether informed consent to the proposed treatment – chemotherapy, has been given. Informed consent and truth-telling are clearly closely connected in the issues they raise.

The UKCC document on Accountability (UKCC, 1989) states that the motivation for withholding information must never be that it is in the interests of the professional rather than the patient. The harmful results of withholding information are clear in the distrust and distress subsequently felt by this patient. It is unjustifiable both according to the autonomy principle and in terms of what is in the patient's interests.

Here the nurse does take it upon herself to pick up the pieces and to give the patient the information that she has not had. Is this acceptable? It has been suggested above that the nurse should try other courses of action before attempting to intervene with the patient. In this case, however, she is not giving absolutely new information so much as explaining what has previously been told, in a roundabout way. In this way, nurses frequently interpret what a doctor has said and give explanations to patients about specific procedures. Thus, they are contributing to the provision of informed consent.

Conclusion

In nursing the adult it is clear that autonomy, and informed consent, are central. It has been argued that in the case of competent adults the presumption must be that they are the best judges of what is in their own interests.

To discriminate against certain patients on the grounds of irrelevant characteristics is unjust. Giving patients worse treatment because they are felt to be manipulative or sexually threatening is unjustifiable because it fails to look behind the behaviour of the individual in an attempt to discover the real needs of that patient.

References

American Nurses' Association (1985) *Code for Nurses with Interpretive Statements* (Kansas: ANA).

Assey, J. L. and Herbert, J. M. (1983) 'Who is the seductive patient?' *American Journal of Nursing*, vol. 83, pp. 531–2.

Bandman, E. L. and Bandman, B. (1985) *Nursing Ethics in the Life Span* (Norwalk: Appleton-Century-Crofts).

Bell, N. K. (1981) 'Whose autonomy is at stake?' *American Journal of Nursing*, vol. 81, pp. 1170–2.

Collier, J. (1989) *The Health Conspiracy: How Doctors, the Drug Industry and the Government Undermine Our Health* (London: Century Hutchinson).

Faulder, C. (1985) *Whose Body Is It?: The Troubling Issue of Informed Consent* (London: Virago).

Gallie, W. B. (1955–6) 'Essentially contested concepts', *Proceedings of the Aristotelian Society*, vol. LVI, pp. 167–98.

Gillon, R. (1985) 'Autonomy and consent', in M. Lockwood (ed.) *Moral Dilemmas in Modern Medicine*, pp. 111–25 (Oxford: Oxford University Press).

Guardian, 'What should a patient know?', 1 March 1984.

Guardian, 'Scarman backs informed consent', 22 February 1985.

Holder, A. R., Lewis, R. and J. W. (1981) 'Informed consent and the nurse', *Nursing Law & Ethics*, vol. 2, pp. 1–2, 8.

Hull, R. T. (1982) 'Dealing with sexism in nursing and medicine', *Nursing Outlook*, vol. 30, pp. 89–94.

McMorrow, M. E. (1981) 'The manipulative patient', *American Journal of Nursing*, vol. 81, pp. 1188–90.

Mill, John Stuart (1859) *On Liberty*, in *Three Essays* (1975) pp. 5–141 (Oxford: Oxford University Press).

Muff, J. (1988) 'Of images and ideals: a look at socialization and sexism in nursing', in A. Hudson-Jones (ed.) *Images of Nurses: Perspectives from History, Art and Literature* (Philadelphia: University of Pennsylvania Press).

Muyskens, J. L. (1982) *Moral Problems in Nursing: a Philosophical Investigation* (Totowa: Rowman & Littlefield).

Pellegrino, E. D. (1979) 'Towards a reconstruction of medical morality: the primacy of the act of profession and the fact of illness', *Journal of Medicine and Philosophy*, vol. 4, pp. 32–56.

United Kingdom Central Council for Nursing, Midwifery and Health Visiting (1984) *Code of Professional Conduct for the Nurse, Midwife and Health Visitor*, 2nd ed. (London: UKCC).

United Kingdom Central Council for Nursing, Midwifery and Health Visiting (1989) *Exercising Accountability: A Framework to Assist Nurses, Midwives and Health Visitors to Consider Ethical Aspects of Professional Practice* (London: UKCC).

Veatch, R. M. (1990) 'Physician–patient relationship will change', *Medical Ethics Advisor*, vol. 6, pp. 2–3.

Williams, B. (1969) 'The idea of equality', in J. Feinberg (ed.) *Moral Concepts* (Oxford: Oxford University Press).

Young, G. (1981) 'A woman in medicine: reflections from the inside', in H. Roberts (ed.) *Women, Health and Reproduction* (London: Routledge & Kegan Paul).

6·Nursing the unborn and newborn

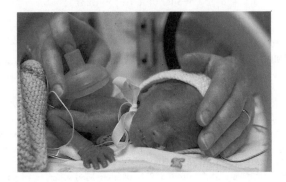

Introduction

The issues raised in the context of nursing the unborn and newborn are sometimes agonising ones. They frequently concern matters of life and death, and many problems, such as that of abortion, have generated and continue to generate much discussion. What we shall try to do in this chapter is to throw light on new developments, and on the ways in which the issues specifically affect nurses. The issue of abortion is one that arises for every health professional and every thinking person. It is nurses, however, who may have to handle a dead foetus, and to care for women even if, in some cases, they disapprove of their reasons for having an abortion.

Thinking about the issues

Nurses may have special problems to face, and it is important that they are aware of current legislation and that they know what their position is on the issues that are common to everyone. There is a recognised right to refuse to participate in some procedures if individuals consider them to be unethical (Abortion Act, 1967, s.4). The Code of Conduct (clause 7) holds that the nurse shall 'make known to an appropriate person or authority any conscientious objection which may be relevant to professional practice' (UKCC, 1984).

But, as Bandman and Bandman point out, nurses should identify their position on such matters before they are actually confronted with them (Bandman and Bandman, 1985, p. 134). There is always the possibility, of course, that a nurse may change her mind when assisting at such a procedure, but it is clearly preferable to have thought about the ethical issues beforehand.

So, let us look at the relevant issues in nursing the unborn and newborn.

Who is the patient?

In the context of the unborn and newborn, there is often a problem in determining who is the patient: who is it that is receiving care. In nursing a pregnant woman, for example, is there only one patient, or two? If one, is it the mother or the foetus? If two, which should take priority when there is a clash of interests?

Although there are grounds for saying that, in the case of other client groups, the boundaries of care also extend beyond an individual patient to, for example, partners and children, the question of other interested parties is particularly pressing in the context of the unborn and newborn. This is partly because the latter are never in a position to speak for themselves. In their case, we cannot follow the principle of respect for autonomy, because they do not have the capacity for autonomy. But if we simply follow the principle of respecting the autonomy of the adults involved, we may fail to protect the interests of the unborn and newborn.

What we need to do is to look at the different interests and issues that may be involved in this context, in order to assess how the dilemmas that arise can be resolved.

Adults

Control of fertility

There are several ways in which the interests of adults may be at stake in relation to the unborn and newborn. For women, in particular, the control of their own fertility continues to be an issue. There is a demand for efficient contraception, and for access to abortion in the case of contraceptive failure. This is a central aspect of feeling in control of their own lives and bodies.

For obvious reasons, this is an issue that affects men less, but it does not follow that they have no interests at all in the matter. Cases of fathers attempting to prevent their partners from aborting a foetus show that they may have very strong feelings, giving rise to a conflict of interests (cf. *Observer*, 17 Jan 1988).

Apart from the problem of *preventing* unwanted pregnancy, another aspect of control of fertility concerns those who are infertile and unhappy about it. Certain technologies, such as artificial insemination and *in vitro* fertilisation, have made it possible for people who were previously unable to have a child, to do so. Issues that have commonly been raised in this context include whether or not infertility should be 'treated' at the public expense and on what criteria patients should be considered suitable for treatment. For example, should single women be granted artificial insemination by donor or should the service be available only to married couples? How far, in other words, should we go in trying to satisfy demand? Nurses, particularly those who are likely to work in the facilities offering this service, should be aware of these issues, just as the profession as a whole has the responsibility to put forward its views in the public debates.

Genetic control

The second issue which is going to become increasingly contentious is to what extent attempts should be made to control the genetic quality of children. Decisions about quality may be made at various stages: genetic counselling may be offered to potential parents; screening of the foetus (by ultrasound, chorion villus sampling, or amniocentesis) may be followed by an offer to abort the foetus; in some cases handicapped newborn infants have been allowed to die (Kuhse and Singer, 1985, pp. 1–17).

In both these areas, as far as the parents are concerned, nurses may be dealing with people who are experiencing profound emotions concerned with their desire to have a child, and with their fears about possible handicap. How far should their wishes in this area be respected?

The answer to this question will depend, in part, on what view is taken about the status of the unborn and newborn – embryos, foetuses and infants – and, in part, on what moral principles are applied.

Embryos

Parliament has now voted to permit experiments on human embryos up to a period of 14 days after fertilisation. The experiments, it is argued, will be of help both in the advancement of treatment for infertility and in screening for genetic disease.

In the continuing debates on the issue, questions arise which seem to lack answers. There is a difference of opinion, for example, about whether or not embryos can be defined as human beings or persons. In one sense, they are clearly human beings, in that they are living beings, and they are part of the human species. But, it is argued by many that we owe respect only to *persons*, and while they may have the potential for personhood they are certainly not actual persons.

On this view, to be a human being is not necessarily to be a person. So when does personhood start? Some argue that being a person is a matter of possessing certain *characteristics*, such as rationality, language or moral capacities. On these criteria, even infants and some adults would not qualify.

Others point to a particular *event* which marks the beginning of personhood, such as birth, but it is not clear why movement from one place (inside the womb) to another place (outside) should make such a difference.

In the case of the embryo, much has been made of the 'primitive streak', a heaping up of cells at one end of the embryo which is said to mark the beginning of the development of the individual (Warnock, 1985, para. 11.22). It is not necessarily claimed that the primitive streak is the beginning of personhood, but that it is the beginning of an identifiable individual with the potential to develop into a person. Before that point, it is argued, we do not know whether we are dealing with an organism that has the potential to develop into one person, or two, or neither. Up to 14 days, the 'pre-embryo', as it is sometimes called, may split into twins or may form nothing more than an abnormal growth known as a hydatiform mole (cf. Harris, 1990, p. 68).

The view that no individual exists until the primitive streak does not have universal support. After all, those pre-embryos, in which the primitive streak appears, do have the potential to develop into persons, even if we do not know which they are.

What is clear about the issues is that there is considerable disagreement. The position we shall take is that this question cannot be settled; that, as the Warnock report held in relation to the embryo:

> Although the questions of when life or personhood begin appear to be questions of fact susceptible of straightforward answers, we hold that the answers to such questions in fact are complex amalgams of factual and moral judgments. Instead of trying to answer these questions directly we have therefore gone straight to the question of *how it is right to treat the human embryo.*
>
> (Warnock, 1985, para. 11.9)

The question to which Warnock directs us is also a matter of controversy. Let us agree, for the sake of argument, that both the embryo and many (if not all) pre-embryos are human beings and potential persons. Even if we agree on this, there is disagreement about how they ought to be treated.

The principle of autonomy, as suggested above, does not help us, for we are dealing with beings that have no capacity for autonomy.

Some supporters of the principle of the sanctity of human life argue that the life of the embryo has absolute value from the moment of fertilisation and that it is wrong to take its life. Those of a consequentialist outlook, on the other hand, may say that we have to consider what will lead to the best consequences, and that while the life of an embryo has value, it does not have absolute value, such that it can override all other considerations. For example, we should consider the value of the embryo's life, and the effect of its existence on others, along with the potential benefits of experiments.

These issues become sharper in the consideration of foetuses.

Foetuses

Abortion

The status of the foetus is as difficult to resolve as that of the embryo. Again, it is not a simple matter of fact, but depends on what value we put on foetal life. However much we know about the facts of foetal development, controversy will continue.

This becomes obvious if we allow, once again for the sake of argument, that the foetus is a person, or at least a potential person. For some, this settles the issue, but for others it does not. It depends on what ethical theory we apply.

As a rights issue, it is normally seen as a clash between the right of the foetus to life, and the right of the mother to choose what happens to and in her own body. The problem is, how can we judge what should happen in the case of such a clash of rights? Which right should take priority?

It is at this point that the consequentialist argues that rights theory cannot answer this question. We need to have some way of weighing up the different interests involved, and of seeing what will lead to the greatest satisfaction of interests. The interests to be taken into consideration include not only those of the mother and foetus, but also other family members, the health care delivery team and society as a whole.

The fact that the majority of people are willing to accept abortion for severe cases of genetic handicap shows a widespread tendency to give some weight to consequences. For it would be difficult, on a rights approach, to argue that a handicapped foetus has less right of life than a 'normal' one. Rather, the argument looks at what life would be like for that child and its family, if an abortion is not carried out.

Once the importance of considering the consequences for the interests of all is admitted in such cases, it is difficult to avoid it in other cases. This applies not simply to cases of abortion but also to the embryo. As John Harris has pointed out, for example, if abortion of foetuses is accepted for the sake of the health of the mother, it is inconsistent to refuse to countenance embryo experiments, which could help many more people (Harris, 1989, p. 88).

The question about the moral acceptability of abortion, however, takes place both at the individual level, concerning particular abortion decisions, and at the social level, concerning what social policy should be. At both levels the issue can be dealt with by considering the consequences for the interests involved. One consequentialist argument for a liberal abortion policy is that a more restrictive one would do more harm overall, because women, if denied legal ones, will continue to seek abortions illegally, not only adding to their distress but also endangering their health. To approve of a liberal social policy, however, does not commit one to approving of particular abortion decisions. As Linda Clarke points out, 'one can be pro-choice but not necessarily pro-abortion' (Clarke, 1989, p. 166).

Nor does it commit one to approving of every kind of abortion. It has recently been argued in the USA that if one is entitled to seek an abortion, one is also entitled to demand that the termination be performed without any attempt to preserve the life of the foetus. In other words, in a post-viability abortion, it is not sufficient that the woman in question be relieved of the pregnancy. Nan Hunter has argued that one is harmed by 'coerced parenthood', by the existence (anywhere) of a genetically related offspring whom one does not want (Hunter, 1989, p. 131).

It is difficult, from a consequentialist perspective, to sympathise with this view. The claim is that one's interests may be sufficiently harmed by the mere existence of another person (rather than by their occupancy of one's body) that their death is justified when it is not a necessary consequence of being freed from the pregnancy. But it is not at all clear how an interest in not having a genetically related offspring can outweigh that offspring's interest in life.

Foetal transplants

A further recent development has been the use of aborted foetal material, in brain tissue transplants, for patients suffering from Parkinson's disease. This is found distasteful by many.

The issue is clouded by its link with abortion. Anti-abortionists clearly have a reason for opposing this technique. From a consequentialist perspective, however, if an abortion has occurred, and there is certain material in existence that could be used to help another to regain health, it would seem wrong *not* to use it. Problems would arise if people were persuaded or coerced into having abortions *in order to* provide material for transplant. It is not only anti-abortionists who might think that the practice could lead to a larger number of abortions being performed.

The Polkinghorne Report which pronounced on this question recommended that great care should be taken to separate the decision relating to abortion, and decisions relating to the subsequent use of foetal tissue (Polkinghorne, 1989, para. 6.4.).

If the decisions are kept separate, then the question amounts to this: given that there is foetal tissue available, should it be put to a potentially good use or not?

Nurses need to be aware of the issues in order to be able to decide whether or not they wish to participate. The Code of Practice issued by Polkinghorne states:

> No member of the medical or nursing staff should be under any duty to participate in research or therapy involving the foetus or foetal tissues if he or she has conscientious objection. This right of non-participation does not extend to the prior or subsequent care of a patient thus treated.
>
> (Polkinghorne, 1989, s.5)

If they do participate, nurses have an obligation, as do other health care staff, to see that the guidelines are observed.

Foetal therapy and maternal–foetal conflict

Issues of conflict between the foetus's interest in life and the mother's interest in choice, in the context of abortion are long-standing. What is *new* is an increasing tendency to regard the foetus as a patient. This is not only because of techniques, such as ultrasound, which enable the monitoring of foetal development, but also because there have been cases of prenatal treatment such as an operation on the heart of a foetus (*Guardian*, 1 February 1990).

Apart from possible concerns about resource implications arising from an increase in foetal treatment, problems arise over the fact that the foetus is within the body of another, whose body necessarily has to be invaded in order to treat the foetus. Who is the patient in such cases? This is a particularly difficult question for those who see the nurse's role as that of an advocate. What if the mother objects to foetal therapy? This leads to a clash between the interests of the foetus, in life and health, and the mother's interest in respect for her autonomy, which is very difficult to resolve. In the USA, similar conflicts have led to forced caesarians (Annas, 1982) and post-birth prosecutions of women for child neglect (Annas, 1986).

As Ruth Macklin argues, it is unlikely to be profitable to look at the question in terms of a conflict of rights between the mother and the foetus – for example, the right to choose versus the right to life. Rights are adversarial and 'the birthing process should be a source of joy and cooperation' (Macklin, 1984, p. 222). She advocates a consequentialist analysis for this problem too, in which we try to assess the effects on the interests of the different people involved, and aim for the best result.

In this context, however, the results are uncertain. Foetal therapy is still so new that it is frequently unclear how beneficial the results will be to the foetus. Mistakes may also be made in screening the foetus for defects. The risks to the mother, however, are fairly clear, including not only those involved in the treatment but also the indignity in being forced against her will to take part. On the other hand, it may be felt that the foetus's interest in life, though uncertain, outweighs other interests.

Because they feel that the foetus is at a disadvantage, being unable to speak in defence of its interests, some writers have considered the possibility of an advocate specifically for the foetus (e.g. Macklin, 1984, p. 213), but this argument presents problems. The general difficulties related to the notion of advocacy have been considered earlier. However, in this context, as Macklin points out, what if both physician and parents wanted the therapy, but the advocate was against it? In that case, how much weight should be given to the advocate's view?

Problems may arise for nurses if they disagree with particular decisions in these cases. For example, they may disapprove of a mother's decision to refuse therapy for a foetus, or they may be shocked by the treatment of a mother undergoing a forced caesarian. The problem of being clear about one's own values in such situations is followed by that of accepting the limitations, in many cases, to what one can do about them. This point is relevant to all the dilemmas we are looking at in this chapter.

Infants

Some people feel that an infant has a status that is totally different from that of a foetus. In an obvious sense, it has joined society by becoming a visible member of it. Others, however, feel that there is no difference in principle between a being that is inside the womb and one that is outside it: it is simply a matter of geography. This view is supported by the increasingly earlier viability limit and techniques for examining the foetus while it is still in the womb.

It is difficult to accept, then, that the status of the newborn infant is significantly different from that of the foetus. Again, however, the facts do not solve any moral issues. Once more it is a moral question we have to answer, about how infants should be treated.

There are two main problem areas here: the first concerns care in the neonatal intensive care unit (NICU) for babies of very low birthweights, and the second concerns allowing severely handicapped babies to die.

NIC units and low birthweight babies

Marshall and Kasman have documented the phenomenon of burnout in the neonatal intensive care unit (Marshall and Kasman, 1980). This is partly due to facts of life that have always been with us, namely the difficulty of coming to terms with the death of infants and the feelings of failure that follow. But, Marshall and Kasman point out that recent developments have made the problem of burnout worse. The constant arrival of new treatments threatens the nurse's sense of competence. Also, we are now seeing a new kind of patient in NICUs: the chronic patient. Whereas in the past babies with very low birthweights would have died within a week, they may now survive but develop chronic lung disease. Their long-term prospects are also uncertain. Ruth Macklin argues:

> In the case of many premature and low birthweight
> infants . . . the decision to treat aggressively may result in
> preserving the life of an individual who will be severely
> damaged, possessing such a poor quality of life that either
> prolonged suffering or inability to relate to other human beings
> is the outcome . . . .. Applying a utilitarian calculus, we would
> most likely conclude that the early death of such infants
> produces the most favorable consequences for all who stand to
> be affected.

> (Macklin, 1984, p. 218)

Against this kind of reasoning, as Bandman and Bandman point out, nurses may see themselves as advocates for the helpless infants (Bandman and Bandman, 1985, p. 144). Some may want to give overriding priority to their interest in life. But Macklin's point is that the consequence of early death is best for all, including the infants themselves. The question of the lengths to which we should go to preserve such infant life is a question that faces society as a whole, but which arises with particular urgency for nurses working in NIC units.

Severely handicapped infants

Related issues arise when severely handicapped infants are rejected by their parents. There have been one or two well publicised cases of this, such as the John Pearson case in the UK and the Baby Doe case in the USA (cf. Kuhse and Singer, 1985, pp. 1–17).

The clash between consequentialist and other values comes into play once more. Should we take the view that an infant, however severely handicapped, has a life that should be protected and prolonged indefinitely? Or should we think about the consequences, for the infant, its family, and society, of the infant's continued existence?

Those who take the former view run into difficulties over anencephalic babies, who have no potential for a life of any quality. Some have suggested that anencephalics should be used as sources of organs for babies who do have such potential (*Guardian*, 1 February 1990). There are clearly consequentialist arguments for this, and it may help some parents to feel that their baby's life, doomed and limited though it was, would not have been in vain.

Acts and omissions

Suppose a decision is taken, for whatever reason (perhaps from compassion), that an infant's life should not be extended, what does this imply? Let us imagine, for example, that parents reject the baby. It is not always the case, of course, that the parents' rejection of the baby entails its death, but in some cases it does, where they refuse permission for a life-prolonging intervention. In some cases like this, health care professionals have brought about or hastened the death of the babies in question by not treating them, and sometimes by not even feeding them, thus relying on the principle of acts and omissions, that it is worse to kill than to allow to die. Reading the story of John Pearson's slow death, however, gives us further reasons for refusing to accept this principle (Kuhse and Singer, 1985, pp. 1–11). Such a death is arguably far more cruel (or, it has worse consequences) than a quick and painless death. The judge, however, in the Arthur case, relied on a distinction between murder and setting the conditions in which death is allowed to occur (Kuhse and Singer, 1985, p. 7).

The law would not, of course, accept such a position with regard to a baby that was not handicapped in any way. Mr Justice Farquharson's remarks applied to an infant both irreversibly disabled and rejected by its parents. What the decision tells us is that the judge agreed with the doctor and the parents that it would be better for all concerned if the baby was dead. If that decision is made, why not initiate that death as quickly and humanely as possible?

One argument for not allowing this to happen is that it will lead to less respect for the lives of handicapped people in general. Kuhse and Singer, however, have assessed evidence from other societies where infanticide is practised and have concluded that the killing of newborn infants does not necessarily have unwelcome implications for the manner in which other people in society are treated (Kuhse and Singer, 1985, pp. 98–117). This is not because infants suddenly turn into persons at a particular point, but it does show that, psychologically speaking, a sharp distinction can be drawn between our responses to infanticide and to the taking of other forms of human life.

If it is thought that infanticide is morally permissible in some circumstances, the question arises as to whether the practice should remain secret and hidden as it is now, or whether it should be open, a social policy regulated by law, which would have to stipulate a time limit, as it does for abortion and embryo research.

Who decides?

Some of the most difficult issues in nursing the unborn and newborn concern decision-making. It is all very well, it might be argued, for us to discuss what should happen in cases such as those outlined above, but we are not the ones who are going to have to live with the results of those decisions on a daily basis.

Let us take maternal–foetal conflict. Clearly, the person most closely affected, apart from the foetus, is the mother. Because of this, even if we think that, in a particular case, a woman might be wrong to refuse therapy for her foetus, a policy of allowing the woman to decide seems preferable as leading to the best consequences overall. Otherwise, as Nelson and Milliken point out, we should be accepting the undermining of autonomy and bodily integrity for a particular group of patients, i.e. mothers (Nelson and Milliken, 1988, p. 1065). The foetus has not developed the capacity for autonomy, but the mother has. The undermining of patient autonomy for one group may have undesirable consequences for respect of patient autonomy in other areas.

In such cases the father's interests, as we have noted, are not as closely involved as those of the mother. In the case of embryo research, however, this is not so. The embryo in the laboratory is not linked to either parent any more than to the other. Both have contributed their gametes. In this area, then, it makes sense for both gamete donors to be asked for their consent to the embryo's use.

When we turn to newborn infants, the situation is more complicated. There has been some evidence of a desire to respect parents' wishes in cases like that of John Pearson. From a consequentialist point of view, as in decisions about abortion and foetal therapy, the best result may be achieved by letting parents decide. Some would object to this on the grounds that the reasoning powers of parents in such dilemmas are clouded by distress. Should the doctor or an ethics committee make the decision? But, just as the parents' judgment may be affected by their closeness to the situation, that of others may be affected by distance from it. It is not, in an obvious sense, anyone else's tragedy.

One thing is clear, the nurse is unlikely to be an ultimate decision-maker, and may not only profoundly disapprove but also have the distressing task of, for example, comforting a dying infant. In one or two cases it has been suggested that it was nurses who played a major part in bringing such incidents to public attention (Robertson, 1981, pp. 5, 7). A principal theme of the cases in this chapter is the way in which nurses come to feel alienated from the work in which they are involved.

The cases

'Getting rid of' a defective foetus

❝ We'll get rid of it for you ❞

Whilst working in an antenatal clinic a pregnant woman, who badly wanted a baby, came in with her husband for a routine check-up. On palpation the doctor was not happy with the growth of the baby and sent the woman for a scan. I was with her when she had her scan. Her husband was also present. The radiographer said 'Oh, there's something not quite right here – I'll get the doctor'. I was sent to ask the consultant to come and look at the scan. She did this and very quickly said: 'this baby is obviously not growing properly – come in to the ward next week and we'll get rid of it for you'. Both the woman and her husband were devastated. They were given no choice as to whether or not to terminate the pregnancy. I tried to comfort them but they just wanted to get out of the room and go home.

Commentary

Let us, first, set aside the issue of the status of the foetus in this case. We are given no information as to the degree of its handicap or its stage of development. This case illustrates the point made earlier that nursing the unborn also includes caring for the parents, or would-be parents, at a stage of their lives that is marked by deep emotions.

To the doctor, the issue may have seemed clear-cut: the foetus was not growing properly, and it would be better for all concerned if the pregnancy was terminated.

The case shows, however, that the moral issues do not stop with a decision that a particular termination is or is not justified.

The principle of respect for persons includes showing some consideration for their feelings. The language used here shows none. To employ the term 'get rid of it' to a pregnant woman desperate for a baby is, to say the least, thoughtless.

The nurse is left in the position of 'picking up the pieces'. She does see the importance of a different approach, and also adds that the couple was not given any choice. Should they have been?

We have argued that, while it is not the case that the wish of the parents is the only consideration, in general the best results will be gained if they are allowed to choose. It may be that, in the doctor's view, no option other than a termination was a viable one, but the facts could have been explained to the parents in such a way that they themselves came to see the necessity of this course of action. This would have allowed them to maintain some sense of control over their own lives in the midst of their personal tragedy.

Disagreeing with an abortion decision

‹ She eventually aborted the foetus into the bed pan ›

A young girl came in to have a prostaglandin termination. I had no firm views against termination when I entered nursing, and did not request to be allowed to avoid a ward where terminations were being carried out. I had also witnessed several terminations before seeing this particular one. This one, however, greatly upset me. The whole moral issue of maintaining life arose for me when this girl of about 15 or 16 years of age was attached to the prostaglandin pump. When she eventually aborted the foetus into the bed pan I just looked at it. It was a boy, all fingers, toes, two arms, two legs, a little hair on his head. The girl didn't want to look. There was a staff nurse present who clamped the cord. But I felt very sad inside, thinking of the women on the ward on continuous bed rest, having had previous miscarriages and desperately wanting children. I found it quite hard being civil to the girl in the morning.

Commentary

It has been argued above that nurses should think out their moral position before they are required to face particular situations. This case, however, suggests that this does not always work. Situations will arise which surprise or even shock the nurse in the emotions to which they give rise. No serious moral dilemma arises here: the nurse is clear about how she should behave, but there is an illustration here of how difficult it may be to separate private disapproval of a patient's choice and treating the patient with respect.

Falsely telling parents their premature baby was stillborn

‹ I turned to see the baby breathing and whimpering like a puppy ›

It was my first span of night duty. A woman, 24 to 25 weeks pregnant, was admitted for a urinary tract infection. She was about 32 years old, happily married, and had been trying for a baby for about 10 years.

At the beginning of the shift, our report said that this lady was having a bright red loss and severe regular pains. Seeing her, it was obvious that she was in early labour. Her husband was with her.

The senior registrar was called and arrived just in time to deliver a premature baby. He took the 'dead' baby into the sluice and placed it on the draining board. The distressed parents were told that their baby daughter was stillborn. The father asked to see her. One of the other nurses refused to handle the baby herself but agreed to accompany me while I performed offices on her. On entering the sluice, we heard a feeble cry, and turned to see the baby breathing and whimpering like a puppy. I ran down the ward to inform the doctor, whose reaction was 'I know nurse, but it won't live long!' The baby lived for one and a half hours on the draining board during which time I was stalling for time with the father who was anxious to see her. To this day those parents believe their girl was stillborn.

Commentary

Two issues arise in connection with this case. The first is whether any effort should have been made to prolong the baby's life; the second is whether the parents should have been told the truth. These issues are connected in that the decision made about the first leads naturally to that made about the second, but, as far as the nurse is concerned, she has far more freedom of action with regard to the second than the first.

Let us suppose that the doctor made the decision from a consequentialist perspective, and that the reasoning took the following form. The baby's chances of survival were minimal: she was very premature. Any attempt to extend her life would only prolong the distress of the parents, without any prospect of sufficient benefit to make this worthwhile. So, from a consequentialist perspective, the answer to the first question seems to be 'no'.

That being so, the truth has to be concealed from the parents, for if they knew what was really happening this would certainly increase their suffering. Given the hopeless outlook, the best results for them would be gained by leaving the baby to die and keeping quiet about the circumstances.

One obvious fault with such an analysis is that it ignores the position of the nurse. She is faced with the task of keeping up the deception and delaying the father, while having to deal with her own emotions concerning the baby's fate. What are the long-term consequences for nurse–patient relationships if nurses are expected to behave like that?

Second, if we include long-term consequences as well as short-term ones, is it clear that in the long run it is best for the parents to be denied the truth? Might they not ultimately adjust to the knowledge of what had actually happened?

If we turn away from thinking about the consequences of actions to other considerations, some would take the view that, since all life is of value, every attempt should have been made to save the baby. As far as the deception is concerned, an objection to this is that it does not show respect for the parents. An assumption is made that they cannot cope with the truth about the fate of their own daughter; that to lie to them is in their best interests.

The nurse is not responsible for initiating this deception, but should she go along with it? The case description suggests that her view is that the action taken was not in their best interests, and thus that she lied because she felt she had to. If so, then it is arguable that she should not comply, but it is, of course, for her to make the decision.

Conclusion

In the case of the unborn and newborn, some of the most difficult conflicts occur because inevitably the interests of parents, in addition to those of foetuses and infants, are at stake. It appears that the principle of autonomy is only of limited value in the nursing dilemmas discussed here because, while adults have a capacity for autonomy, foetuses and infants do not. Although they may be said to have interests, the nurse frequently has to try to weigh up competing ones, in order to decide what will lead to the best result.

References

Annas, G. J. (1982) 'Forced cesareans: the most unkindest cut of all', *Hastings Center Report*, vol. 12, pp. 16–17, 45.

Annas, G. J. (1986) 'Women as fetal containers', *Hastings Center Report*, vol. 16, pp. 13–14.

Bandman, E. L. and Bandman, B. (1985) *Nursing Ethics in the Life Span* (Norwalk: Appleton-Century-Crofts).

Clarke, L. (1989) 'Abortion: a rights issue?', in R. Lee and D. Morgan, *Birthrights: Law and Ethics at the Beginning of Life*, pp. 155–71 (London: Routledge).

Guardian, 'Doctors who operated on foetus consider ethics of technology', 1 February 1990.

Harris, J. (1989) 'Should we experiment on embryos?' in R. Lee and D. Morgan, *Birthrights: Law and Ethics at the Beginning of Life*, pp. 85–95 (London: Routledge).

Harris, J. (1990) 'Embryos and hedgehogs: on the moral status of the embryo', in A. Dyson and J. Harris (eds), *Experiments on Embryos*, pp. 65–81 (London: Routledge).

Hunter, N. D. (1989) 'Time limits on abortion', in S. Cohen and N. Taub (eds) *Reproductive Laws for the 1990s*, pp. 129–53 (Clifton, N. J.: Humana Press).

Kuhse, H. and Singer, P. (1985) *Should the Baby Live?: The Problem of Handicapped Infants* (Oxford: Oxford University Press).

Macklin, R. (1984) 'The ethics of fetal therapy', in J. M. Humber and R. T. Almeder (eds) *Biomedical Ethics Reviews*, pp. 205–33 (Clifton, N. J.: Humana Press).

Marshall, R. E. and Kasman, C. (1980) 'Burnout in the neonatal intensive care unit', *Pediatrics*, vol. 65, pp. 1161–65.

Nelson, L. J. and Milliken, N. (1988) 'Compelled treatment of pregnant women: life, liberty and law in conflict', *Journal of the American Medical Association*, vol. 259, pp. 1060–6.

Observer, 'Abortion case father raises campus baby', 17 January 1988.

Polkinghorne, J. (Chairman) (1989) *Code of Practice on the Use of Fetuses and Fetal Material in Research and Treatment* (London: HMSO).

Polkinghorne, J. (Chairman) (1989) *Review of the Guidance on the Research Use of Fetuses and Fetal Material* (London: HMSO).

Robertson, J. A. (1981) 'Dilemma in Danville', *Hastings Center Report*, vol. 11, pp. 5–8.

United Kingdom Central Council for Nursing, Midwifery and Health Visiting (1984) *Code of Professional Conduct for the Nurse, Midwife and Health Visitor*, 2nd ed. (London: UKCC).

Warnock, M. (1985) *A Question of Life: The Warnock Report on Human Fertilisation and Embryology* (Oxford: Blackwell).

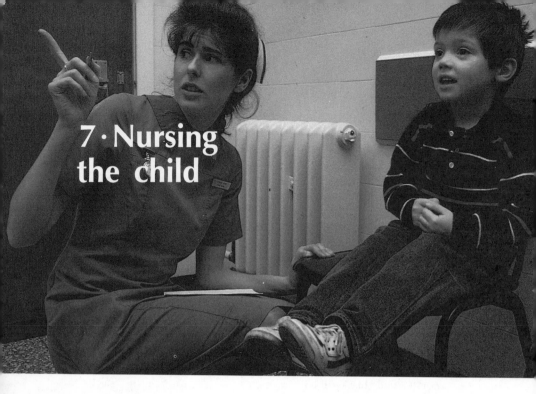

7 · Nursing the child

Introduction

The concept of childhood is relatively new in terms of social history. From the ancient Greeks until the latter part of the nineteenth century, children were regarded as chattels or the property of their parents. Aristotle in the *Nicomachean Ethics* stated:

> for there can be no injustice in the unqualified sense towards things that are one's own, but a man's chattel, and his child until it reaches a certain age and sets up for itself, are as it were part of himself.

> (Aristotle, 1980, p. 123)

More recently, the great social reformers, such as the Earl of Shaftesbury who 'represented the new social conscience of the mid-nineteenth century' (Baly, 1973, p. 38), did much to highlight the pitiful conditions under which children were raised, made to work and sadly all too soon died. Such conditions have been immortalised by writers such as Dickens and, therefore, need no further exploration here. One should, however, undertand that such conditions arose largely from the view that children were regarded as the property of their parents and, therefore, could be done with, more-or-less, as the parents wished.

A very similar situation prevailed across the Atlantic in the USA. It was Theodore Roosevelt, who, as President in 1909, urged Congress to pass legislation to create a children's bureau which would gather data primarily on the conditions to which children were being subjected, and inform the public of the full facts.

The main opposition to the enactment of such legislation was due to the traditional notion that the family was best placed to determine how children were to be treated. In speaking out against the bill, Senator Joseph Bailey stated, 'We have for 100 years or more left these matters concerning children to the proper authorities, which are mothers, fathers and guardians' (Wilson, 1989).

Today, the situation is very different and great emphasis is placed on the protection of children. Acts and laws have been passed to safeguard children and numerous voluntary bodies, such as the National Society for Prevention of Cruelty to Children (NSPCC), have been established and are primarily concerned with promoting children's interests.

In 1959, the United Nations (UN) published its Declaration of the Rights of the Child, and the 1980s has seen increased social concern with regard to child abuse generally and child sexual abuse in particular.

These changing attitudes and influences towards the treatment and raising of children has meant that the State is more willing to intervene on behalf of children and professionals, from a variety of backgrounds, come into closer contact with a greater number of children. These professionals include health care professionals generally and nurses in particular. Therefore, it is somewhat surprising that, other than those issues concerning neonates, relatively little is to be found in the UK literature about the moral concerns raised when nursing older children.

One fundamental principle in children's nursing is that children are not merely 'miniature adults', they are special and this introduces us to our first issue, that of children as special subjects.

Children as special subjects

A number of situations arise in health care when children are classified as special subjects. The first question that we need to address is, on what morally relevant grounds do children qualify as special subjects? Age alone will not do, as shall be seen in Chapter 8, as it is not a morally relevant characteristic.

The United Nations Declaration of the Rights of Children clearly states that because of physical and mental immaturity, children need special protection and care (UN, 1959). This immaturity means that children cannot fully understand the risks and discomforts that certain procedures would impose and, therefore, they are extremely vulnerable to abuses of power in the child/professional or child/adult relationship.

In an attempt to protect children, the Declaration of Helsinki (1964) demanded proxy consent in the case of a child, by the parent, guardian or legal representative (Declaration of Helsinki, 1964). One needs, however, to exercise a degree of caution in accepting this account, as the term 'children' may be applied equally to those who are two years of age as to those who are fifteen years of age and there are obviously great differences in the levels of understanding between these cases. Kennedy (1985) suggests that to treat all children as a class, having the same status, is to ignore the principle of autonomy as respect for this principle 'involves respect for each person's individuality' (Kennedy, 1985, pp. 32–75).

Children as research subjects

A fundamental question that needs to be addressed is, ought children to be expected to participate in research?

The Declaration of Helsinki recognised a fundamental distinction between therapeutic and non-therapeutic research describing the former as, ' . . . medical research in which the aim is essentially diagnostic or therapeutic for the patient . . . ' and the latter as ' . . . medical research . . . which is purely scientific and without direct diagnostic or therapeutic value to the person subjected to the research' (Declaration of Helsinki, 1964).

Therefore, we need to be aware that, if we allow children to participate, we are undertaking research without the consent of those participating and if we do not, then children become 'therapeutic orphans', that is a class of persons denied the benefits of research (Levine, 1989).

In attempting to solve this fundamental problem, it could be argued that it is relatively easy to justify therapeutic research as indeed many writers have. McCormick (1974) suggests that giving proxy consent to therapeutic interventions does not violate respect for the child as the presumption is that an individual would, if able to, seek his own wellbeing. Freedman, too, argues in favour of the involvement of children on the basis that children have a right to be cared for and, therefore, providing that the research offers no discernible risk, that is the child is protected from harm, then participation is not a problem (Freedman, 1975, pp. 32–9).

Paul Ramsey, although agreeing that research which directly benefits the child concerned may be acceptable, is totally opposed to the notion that it is morally acceptable to involve children in non-therapeutic research. For Ramsey, such research, whether it is with or without risk, is wrong as it negates the principle of respect for persons which demands that it is wrong to touch anyone who has not consented to be touched (Ramsey, 1970, pp. 1–58).

The Declaration of Helsinki requires that those involved in non-therapeutic research must be volunteers and, if one accepts that voluntariness entails free choice that results from understanding and reasoning, it is difficult to imagine how one person, even a parent can volunteer another, namely a child, for a particular purpose. Because of this difficulty, some philosophers have questioned whether it is ever permissible for children, who are unable to give consent on their own behalf, to be involved in research which offers them no direct benefit (Brykcznska, 1989, p. 126).

There are two major arguments against this stance. The first is that participating in research that offers no direct benefit to the subject is a morally good thing and therefore ought to be encouraged in children (Gaylin, 1982; McCormick, 1974; Ackerman, 1979). The second is that the morally relevant characteristic of the research activity is the level of risk that it poses and not whether it is of direct benefit to the participant (Freedman, 1975).

We need to ask, however, if children, as members of a moral community, have to shoulder the responsibilities of the full range of obligations to contribute to the general welfare. Or as Ramsey (1970) suggests, as children are they not exempt from such burdens?

What of Freedman's position, that it is the level of risk that determines whether or not a child should participate in a particular research study? Attempts to determine acceptable levels of risk have been made on both sides of the Atlantic.

In 1981, the US Department of Health and Human Services proposed the following definition. 'Minimal risk means that the risks anticipated in the proposed research are not greater, considering probability and magnitude, than those ordinarily encountered in daily life or during the performance of routine physical or psychological examinations or tests' (DHHS, 1981; *see* US Department of Health and Human Services).

In the UK in 1980, the British Paediatric Association (BPA) accepted the following guidelines which were proposed by a working party and meant to aid ethical committees in their deliberations on the acceptability of research proposals:

- *Negligible risk* – risk less than that run in everyday life;
- *Minimal risk* – risk questionably greater than negligible;
- *More than minimal risk* (BPA, 1980).

Clearly, there are problems in accepting any of these definitions. What are the risks 'run in everyday life' or 'ordinarily encountered in daily life'? Surely this depends on how comparisons are made and on what is to count as everyday life. For example, crossing a busy road, although for many of us part of everyday life, would be far too risky for a child of five years of age, but probably acceptable for a child of twelve or thirteen years of age, as long as the child in question had no significant impairments. Are skiing, flying or absailing to be considered as part of everyday life, which they are for many individuals? Even accepting that most people do not routinely undertake dangerous activities, these definitions assume that we know the risks that the majority of us ordinarily encounter (Kopelman, 1989).

What about children living in certain parts of the world, such as Northern Ireland, where the risks of daily life are undoubtedly greater than they are for those living in rural England? Is it then acceptable that these children can be exposed to greater risks than the latter group? Despite being unjust, this was the very justification offered by those responsible for the hepatitis studies undertaken in the now infamous Willowbrook institution, ' . . . it was apparent that most of the patients at Willowbrook were naturally exposed to hepatitis virus' (Ward *et al*, 1958).

The BPA guidelines give examples of how the different categories of risks might be weighed against potential benefits. For example, research into cystic fibrosis might involve an affected child having a sweat test requiring twice as much sweat as normal. The discomfort to the child may be assessed as being negligible, whereas if a venepuncture was added to this procedure it may move the risk into the minimal category. However, the potential benefit to other children suffering from this disease may be so great as to make these risks and discomforts acceptable. Undoubtedly one can think of research studies of great potential benefit to children generally. For example, taking blood samples from a group of children living close to a motorway network and from a group living in an isolated country village, may tell us a great deal about lead pollution.

However, when one considers the distress experienced by many children by the mere thought of needles and injections, it may be that this study if undertaken on children below a certain age would need to be ruled out because of the fear that it engenders. Harm is not only a physical manifestation but often a psychological one as well.

The concepts of harm and risk are of equal importance, and one needs to be aware that it is possible to be harmed without incurring risks. The BPA guidelines take no account of this factor.

A further example from the BPA guidelines describes how, during an abdominal operation, a renal biopsy might be taken. Such a procedure would constitute a 'more than minimal risk' and so the benefit would need to be considerable for its justification. The benefit cited is that of resolving the problem of transplant rejection which would save the lives of many adults and children in the future and, therefore, according to the BPA ' . . . is of sufficient magnitude to justify the risk' (BPA, 1980).

Bearing in mind that the child undergoing surgery does not suffer from renal disease, is the benefit not too far removed from this particular child to justify such risks? Were this same research to be undertaken on adult subjects, it would require their voluntariness in the giving of informed consent. Should we not at least demand the same standard for children?

Some may argue that informed consent is given by the child's parents, but is this acceptable? In therapeutic research, where the child may be the beneficiary of any experimentation, this may be the case, but it is not a high enough standard to adopt in non-therapeutic research. Parents are especially vulnerable when their child is ill and, as in the Philip Becker case, they may not always decide in the best interests of the child (Annas, 1982, pp. 25–6).

It is worth noting that the BPA, although an organisation presumably concerned with the interests of children, finds it acceptable to allow proxy consent for non-therapeutic procedures. The Medical Defence Union (MDU), which is an organisation concerned solely with the interests of the medical profession, issues advice against such practices. In their publication *Consent to Treatment*, they state, 'The MDU and the DHSS have both been advised that legally no-one can give consent to non-therapeutic treatment of a child except the child himself. If such treatment is proposed, the child should be able to understand fully the nature, purpose and effects of the procedure' (MDU, 1986).

Let us now turn to the issue of children giving consent.

Consent and the child

At some stage, most nurses will be expected to request a patient's consent for specific treatment or surgery and of providing the information on which that consent is based. The notion of consent is an important one in any professional/client relationship, and it is based on the principle of autonomy.

Autonomy is concerned with determining one's own course of action in accordance with one's deliberations, values and aspirations (Chapter 5). Although it is important to remember that autonomy is not an absolute state. In other words, none of us have total freedom in deciding how we are to act in a particular situation as we are all governed by certain constraints. Likewise, the degree to which we can be described as autonomous varies at different times in our lives. For example pain, the influence of drugs, and physical/mental impairment or illness can render us more or less dependent on others.

Childhood involves moving through degrees of autonomy. The very young infant, for example, is totally dependent and gradually as maturity increases so does the ability to make the independent decisions that are part and parcel of the responsibilities of adulthood. Each of us, however, differs considerably in terms of the rate at which we mature and, therefore, the notion of every child becoming autonomous at a specific age is arbitrary and increasingly open to challenge as societal values change. So how are we to judge when a particular child has acquired sufficient autonomy to give consent or indeed to withhold it for a particular treatment?

At this point, it is worth developing this concept of consent as it must certainly mean more than the ability to say 'yes' or 'no'. For consent to be valid it must be given freely, without any duress and the patient must be given an explanation of the nature, purpose and material risks of the proposed procedure (Medical Defence Union, 1986). Consent then becomes informed consent, but we still need to determine the criteria that will enable us to decide whether a particular child is capable of giving 'informed consent' on their own behalf.

Some philosophers claim that it is with the development of rationality alone that one becomes autonomous (Kant, 1963; Paters, 1972), but others such as Gaylin (1982) argue that 'the search for a single test of competency is a search for the Holy Grail' and as such is unhelpful.

Kennedy (1985) explores three approaches that have been used to determine the individual's capacity to consent and these include the content or the outcome of the decision, the status of the individual and the ability to understand or comprehend.

The first of these is problematic as any decision which differs from that of the doctor or the parent could result in the child being declared incompetent, especially when one considers that there is a natural tendency for professionals and parents to believe that 'they know best'.

The second approach, that of the status of the individual is also unhelpful, in the case of children, as it favours the status quo where a minor, by virtue of being a minor, lacks the capacity to consent. Section 8 of the Family Law Reform Act states that the consent of a person aged 16 years or over to medical or dental treatment is valid and, therefore, performance of a procedure does not require the consent of the parent or guardian. Although the Act does not state that children below this age cannot give consent, most practitioners would not proceed with treatment in non-emergency situations without parental consent.

However, is there some essential difference in the ability of a young person to consent at 16 years of age and at 15 and a half years? Even the law recognises varying reference points for minority. For example, one cannot marry without parental consent until the age of 18 years, but one can consent to sexual intercourse at 16 years of age and, as Kennedy points out, a fixed reference point may be necessary for matters of law but it is not necessary for ethical reasoning.

For Kennedy the only valid criterion in judging competence to consent is the ability of the individual concerned to understand the proposed procedure or treatment. Because this test is individually applied, it involves respect for the individual's autonomy (Kennedy, 1985, pp. 32–75).

Brock (1989, p. 181) explores this notion of competence further and indicates that while each of us is competent to undertake some things, others will remain beyond our capacity. Thus, competence is 'task specific'.

Determining competence therefore involves 'matching the capacities of a particular person at a particular time and under particular conditions with the demands of a particular decison-making task' (Brock, 1989, p. 182). He outlines three capacities that should be evident before deciding whether or not a child is competent to consent.

The first of these is the *capacity for understanding and communication* of information which demands that the child must have the cognitive abilities needed to understand the language and concepts relevant to the decision. He also states that they should have sufficient life experience to appreciate what it might be like to be in a particular state or to experience certain conditions.

The second capacity is the *ability to engage in reasoning* which involves making inferences and comparisons as well as weighing and considering the probability of different outcomes.

Finally, the child needs to *be in possession of a set of values* which, when applied to the situation, will enable evaluation of the various benefits and risks. Brock concludes by suggesting that the majority of children have developed these capacities by the age of 14 or 15 years of age and some by the age of 10 to 12 years.

It is at this point, however, that we need to exercise caution because even though a child *is* competent to give consent, it does not automatically follow that we *ought* to allow him to do so. A number of reasons have been proposed as to why we might feel it necessary to ignore the expressed desires of a child. One that is frequently proposed by doctors is that the nature of many medical decisions is complex. When added to the stresses and pain of illness, the complexity often taxes adults, let alone children, to the extent that paternalistic decisions must be made to protect them from the harmful consequences of their choices.

One example often quoted is the case of the Jehovah's Witness. The choice of an adult to refuse a blood transfusion on religious grounds, although difficult, must be accepted on the presumption that the person concerned has considered his or her religious convictions and would rather die than accept the infusion of another person's blood. When the patient is a child, however, even of 12 or 13 years of age, we would not accept that those same religious convictions have been adequately considered to the extent that they alone should be the basis for judging the child's best interests.

However, not all health care decisions are life-threatening and, therefore, the above example is somewhat extreme and as such merely weakens the case for respecting the child's autonomy to consent, rather than refuting it absolutely. Where the decision does not impede the child's development, then it is reasonable that they should be involved in the decision-making and in giving consent. Indeed, it could be argued that this is 'good medicine', as increasing the involvement of the patient often brings with it increased cooperation and compliance with any proposed treatment.

A second and potentially more powerful argument against granting freedom to consent to a child is that of the parents' interests and their rights to decide. Clearly, it is often the parents who have to bear the consequences of treatment involving their children, but surely their claim to decide has to be dependent upon them deciding in their child's best interests. If we return to our family of Jehovah's Witnesses, we would not accept that choosing death rather than a blood transfusion was in the child's best interest and most doctors would take legal action to override the parents' claims. This has been publicised recently in the case of the Cypriot child suffering from leukaemia (*Independent*, 1990).

Mrs Gillick, in her action against Wisbech Health Authority (1984), claimed that she had rights in respect of her children by virtue of being their parent and custodian, as though it were a property issue that was being decided. Children are no longer viewed as the property of their parents and arguably it is wrong to treat them as such.

Society does, however, assign certain responsibilities to parents in raising their children and, in discharging these responsibilities, parents are granted considerable freedom in determining the values and beliefs that they impart to their offspring. This does not mean of course that if a child rejects these values, the parents have the right to impose them. As Ian Kennedy (1985) points out, ' . . . the primary obligation of the parent is to bring the child to an enjoyment of autonomy, as free as possible from constraints on this enjoyment'. The imposition of another's values and beliefs on an individual would be autonomy-reducing and, therefore, not in their best interests.

Robert Holmes suggests that allowing a child authority to make autonomous decisions may be against the interests of the family which is a valued institution within our society and one which, 'carries with it some presumption that others should not intrude into it . . . ' (Holmes, 1989, p. 213).

However, it may be dangerous to assume that any family is an integrated unit with a common set of values. The State frequently intervenes when children are placed 'at risk' as a result of their parents' values, as in cases of neglect, cruelty and child abuse, not to mention ensuring that parents provide for their children's education.

On balance, although health professionals, parents and indeed families as a whole, have legitimate concerns in relation to decisions affecting the wellbeing of the children for whom they care, none of them have independent interests which weigh greater than the child's. The child, in the majority of situations, will bear the major consequences of the choice and, therefore, it is their best interests which must be the principal determinant of any choice.

The cases

Confidentiality and consent to treatment

❝ *She did not want her father to be told of the pregnancy* ❞

While working in the emergency department, I frequently encountered minors seeking treatment without the consent of their parents.
One girl, aged 15 years arrived accompanied by her father. She was
complaining of abdominal pain. After examining her the physician
suspected an ectopic pregnancy which required an immediate
exploratory laparotomy. He asked the girl if she could be pregnant
and she replied that she had missed a period. She then went on to
state that she did not want her father to be told of the pregnancy.
Although the doctor was happy for the girl to sign the consent form
on her own behalf, the head nurse insisted that the father should sign
the consent form, as did the attending surgeon.

The doctor, confronted by his two colleagues, simply wrote
laparotomy on the consent form and explained to the father that
surgery was necessary to remove some blood from his daughter's
abdomen.

The father signed and the girl went to theatre without her father
being made aware that she was pregnant. Although resolved to the
apparent satisfaction of all concerned, I felt that deception had been
practised and no-one had been treated with the respect that they
deserved.

Commentary

Here, we have a young woman almost at the age of consent. Although the
account does not make it clear whether the girl objects to her father
signing the consent form, she objects to him being made aware of her
diagnosis. In other words, she is claiming the right of privacy or
confidentiality over what happens to her body.

If we deny this, we are saying that moral rights, like legal rights,
spring into existence at a particular age and it is patently clear that this
would be an unsatisfactory account of the nature of moral rights. For
example, where would it leave the right to life? In Chapter 10, we shall see
that rights are not absolute, and so we need to consider whether there are
any justifications for overriding them in this particular case.

Perhaps the first questions we ought to ask is, why might this young
woman not wish her father to know that she is pregnant? It may be that
she believes that this knowledge may incur parental wrath or that, on
knowing, her father would think less of her as a daughter. But, is this
sufficient cause to justify deception? By condoning such actions, she may

believe that this is an easy way out of trouble and may, therefore, use such practices in the future to avoid facing up to her failings.

Presumably, if the pregnancy had gone to full term, this girl would have needed and expected the support of her family. One could argue therefore that they have a very real interest in the matter and that they have some interest in avoiding any future unwanted pregnancy. On this view, the parents should be aware of their daughter's activities so that they can advise and counsel her.

Of course, unwanted pregnancy is not the only unfortunate outcome of sexual activity. AIDS and other sexually transmitted diseases may occur and there is much evidence that early sexual intercourse increases the incidence of cervical cancer. These are all reasons as to why parents may have an interest in the type of practices in which their children indulge, as most parents want to avoid unnecessay pain and suffering for their offspring.

A further reason for counselling and persuading this girl from participating in unprotected sex is that she has already had one ectopic pregnancy and a second may result in her future inability to reproduce.

We also need to consider the possible effects of this deceit on the father. If, in the future, he found out that he had been deceived, not only would he be hurt and disappointed in his daughter, thereby possibly injuring family relationships, but he would also lose faith in the medical and health care professionals generally, which may affect his future health care.

Of course, he may not be a very nice father and the girl may well fear a severe beating should he discover the truth. She may also be concerned to protect her partner whom her father may know. Remember that participating in sexual intercourse with a girl under the age of 16 years is a criminal offence, both in this country and in many states in America.

We are not told whether the doctor tried to persuade his patient to be more open or if he offered any counselling about the possible outcomes of her behaviour. This should be the least that he should do, especially as nurses and other doctors know her diagnosis and therefore may inadvertently make the father aware.

On balance, it appears in this case that more harm could result by allowing the deceit and that everyone's best interests would be served by making the father aware of his daughter's predicament.

Refusing treatment

❝ I hated having to spy on her and report her for not eating ❞

As part of my psychiatric experience, I helped care for Angela, a

16-year-old schoolgirl who suffered from anorexia. She weighed under 5 stones when she was first admitted. Her treatment involved her in being totally isolated in a side-ward, not even being allowed to go to the toilet or bathroom. She was watched closely while eating her food and if she did not eat then she was not allowed privileges, like having visitors. If she ate her food, especially high calorie food such as cream cakes, then she was allowed special treats, such as going for short walks, albeit supervised.

Angela's parents had had her admitted against her own expressed wishes. I hated having to spy on her and report her for not eating or drinking her food supplements.

Commentary

Here, we have a girl who under other medical circumstances would have been acknowledged as reaching the age of consent and yet her autonomy has been completely overridden. How can this be justified?

The first point to make is that there is much dispute as to how best to treat anorexia. The regimen described above is one accepted mode of treatment, based on the presumption that the most important principle is to enable the individual to gain weight and then to commence treatment which may involve medication or therapy often involving the family as a whole.

If the stringent restrictions are not imposed, the sufferer frequently resorts to hiding food, vomiting in the toilet or taking excessive doses of laxatives, causing further weight loss and a significant risk to health and life.

No doubt Angela, like most anorectics, would state that she did not wish to die and yet the continued self-denial of food would eventually cause death. Therefore, the treatment is justified on the grounds that Angela's decision not to eat is not a rational decision but is merely symptomatic of her disorder. If she is allowed to refuse treatment then her potential for rationality and autonomy will be denied forever as she will ultimately die. Therefore, it is in her own best interests that the treatment is enforced, especially as the condition does respond to treatment.

The nurse concerned does have some doubts about the way that Angela is treated and experiences a sense of guilt. Nursing does sometimes involve *hard* decisions and practices and this needs to be faced, and support and explanations provided for junior staff. It is, however, not a bad thing that the nurse feels as she does, for overriding an individual's autonomy and enforcing unpleasant treatment is a serious action to take and should only happen in extreme circumstances.

Saving the life of a young person, in a situation such as this, would provide such justification.

Lying to children

    ❜ *Often nurses would lie about an injection not hurting* ❜

During my paediatric experience, I was constantly amazed by the number of qualified nurses and parents who lied to their children. Sometimes the children were very young, such as two or three years of age, but often they were much older, perhaps nine or ten years old.

    Often nurses would lie about an injection or wound dressing not hurting, and parents, especially mothers, would lie about the fact that they were actually going home, saying instead that they were going to the toilet or to see sister. Children were often promised treats that never materialised if they complied or perhaps worse they were 'threatened' with exaggerated accounts of awful things that might happen if they did not comply.

    I asked many nurses why they did this and they always said that it was 'better for the child'. I believe it is always wrong to lie, even to children and it worried me how easily these lies seemed to roll off the tongues of such senior nurses.

Commentary

A frequent justification for lying in health care, as we have already seen, is that it is in the patient's best interest not to be told the truth. Children, however, are often told lies with few or no qualms (Bok, 1979). This happens for many altruistic reasons, such as softening the harshness of the truth or avoiding fear and anxiety as the young are more impressionable and less able to cope with stark facts than are adults. There is nothing new in this. As Bok points out, philosophers such as John Stuart Mill and Grotius both argued that it was quite permissible to lie to children (Bok, 1978, pp. 204–19).

    In part, this may be due to the fact that we all indulge in fantasy and fiction with children. For example, we tell stories about fairies and magical happenings to amuse and encourage youngsters to develop an imagination. There is, however, a world of difference between lying and telling fictional stories, the most important being that stories are not meant to mislead. Children like anyone else, if we are to respect them, should be told the truth except in exceptional circumstances and the giving of an injection or some other unpleasant treatment would hardly count as exceptional.

    When one considers what is to be gained by such lies the answer is very little. For instance, if a child has to have medication by injection and asks if it will hurt, then to say no will only assist the nurse giving the first injection as the child will know that the second one will hurt, and the same applies to changing painful dressings. All that the child has learned is that nurses tell lies and are not to be trusted.

The mother who pretends that she is not going home merely causes her child to distrust her and probably will find that at the next visit, the child will not let her out of his sight. The only other lesson to be gleaned by the child from such behaviour is that it is acceptable to lie as adults do it.

The child gains nothing at all from either experience, the injection still hurts and Mummy has still gone away. Indeed, it could be argued that it is much better to know that something will hurt a little as at least one can prepare onself. As there is nothing in such lies that can benefit the child concerned, it is difficult to see how the nurses can state that it is better for the child.

Surely what they mean is that it saves them the trouble of cajoling, persuading or comforting the child. In other words, it is better for them, but only at that particular moment. It may of course make it all the harder to care for the child on subsequent occasions and can often lead to more and more lies being told.

There are few justifications for nurses to lie to any patient, and children are no exception. Indeed, because children are naturally trusting, it could be argued that it is even more reprehensible to lie to them.

Conclusion

In this chapter we have explored the notion of children as special subjects, particularly in relation to clinical research and we have seen how the application of concepts such as autonomy and informed consent deserve very careful consideration when applied to children and young people.

In children lie society's hope for the future. Whenever we come into contact with the young, to some extent we contribute to the type of persons that they will become. As Brykczynska (1989) states, 'For paediatric nurses, the concern over ethical issues is not a progressive luxury but an integral part of their work'.

References

Ackerman, T. F. (1979) 'Fooling Ourselves with Child Autonomy and Assent in Non-therapeutic Research', *Clinical Research*, vol. 27, pp. 345–48.

Annas, G. J. (1982) 'A Wonderful Case and an Irrational Tragedy: The Phillip Becker Case Continues', *Hastings Center Report*, Feb, pp. 25–6.

Aristotle (1980) *The Nicomachean Ethics*, D. Ross (transl.) (Oxford: Oxford University Press).

Baly, M. E. (1973) *Nursing and Social Change*, pp. 36–45 (London: Heinemann).

Bok, S. (1978) *Lying: Moral Choice in Public and Private Life*, pp. 204–19 (Sussex: Harvester Press).

Bok, S. (1979) 'Lying to Children', *Children's Rights Report*, vol. III, No. 6.

British Paediatric Association (BPA) (1980) 'Guidelines to Aid Ethical Committees Considering Research Involving Children', *Archives of Disease in Childhood*, vol. 55, No. 1, pp. 75–7.

Brock, D. W. (1989) 'Children's Competence for Health Care Decision Making', in L. M. Kopelman and J. C. Moskop (eds), *Children and Health Care: Moral and Social Issues*, pp. 181–212 (Dordrecht: Kluwer Academic Publishers).

Brykczynska, G. M. (ed.) (1989) *Ethics in Paediatric Nursing* (London: Chapman and Hall).

Declaration of Helsinki (1964) Finland.

Freedman, B. (1975) 'A Moral Theory of Informed Consent', *Hastings Center Report*, vol. 5, no. 4, pp. 32–9.

Gaylin, W. (1982) 'The Incompetence of Children: No Longer All or None', *Hastings Center Report*, April, pp. 33–8.

Holmes, R. L. (1989) 'Consent and Decisional Authority in Children's Health Care Decision Making: A Reply to Dan Brock', in L. M. Kopelman and J. C. Moskop (eds), *Children and Health Care: Moral and Social Issues*, pp. 213–19 (Dordrecht: Kluwer Academic Publishers).

Independent 'Doctors to Give Cancer Girl Blood, 16 June 1990.

Kant, I. (1963) *Lectures on Ethics*, Louis Infield (transl.) (New York: Harper and Row).

Kennedy, I. (1985) 'The Doctor, the Pill and the Fifteen-Year-Old Girl', in M. Lockwood (ed.), *Moral Dilemmas in Modern Medicine*, pp. 32–75 (Oxford: Oxford University Press).

Kopelman, L. M. (1989) 'When is the Risk Minimal Enough for Children to be Research Subjects', in L. M. Kopelman and J. C. Moskop (eds), *Children and Health Care: Moral and Social Issues*, pp. 89–99 (Dordrecht: Kluwer Academic Publishers).

Levine, R. J. (1989) 'Children as Research Subjects', in L. M. Kopelman and J. C. Moskop (eds), *Children and Health Care: Moral and Social Issues*, pp. 77–87 (Dordrecht: Kluwer Academic Publishers).

McCormick, R. A. (1974) 'Proxy Consent in the Experimental Situation', *Perspectives in Biology and Medicine*, vol. 18, no. 2, pp. 2–20.

Medical Defence Union (1986) *Consent To Treatment*, p. 16 (London: MDU).

Peters, R. S. (1972) *Ethics and Education*, 3rd ed. (London: George Allen and Unwin).

Ramsey, P. (1970) *The Patient as Person*, pp. 1–58 (New Haven: Yale University Press).

United Nations (UN) (1959) *The Declaration of the Rights of Children* (New York: UN).

US Department of Health and Human Services (1981) 'Final Regulations Amending Basic HHS Policy for the Protection of Human Research Subjects', *Federal Register*, vol. 46, no. 16, Jan 26, pp. 8366–88.

Ward, R. *et al* (1958) 'Infectious Hepatitis: Studies of its Natural History and Prevention', *New England Journal of Medicine*, vol. 258, pp. 407–16.

Wilson, A. L. (1989) 'Development of the US Federal Role in Children's Health Care: A Critical Appraisal', in L. M. Kopelman and J. C. Moskop (eds), *Children and Health Care: Moral and Social Issues* (Dordrecht: Kluwer Academic Publishers).

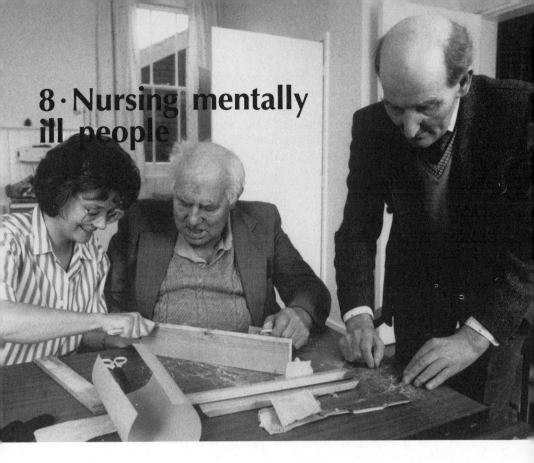

8 · Nursing mentally ill people

Introduction

There has been much controversy about the diagnosis and treatment of mental illness. The 'anti-psychiatry' movement has argued that there is no such thing as mental illness (Szasz, 1962). What we call mental illness, according to such a view, either has a physical cause or it does not. If it does, then it can be counted as real, in so far as it is physical illness. If it does not, then the term 'mental illness' is simply applied to certain forms of behaviour that society finds unacceptable, and finds it convenient to count as illness. We call 'ill' those of whom we disapprove. The abuse of psychiatry to control dissidents in, for instance, the Soviet Union in the pre-Gorbachev era is only an extreme example of this (Bloch, 1984, pp. 322–41).

The fact that minority groups in society are diagnosed as mentally ill more frequently than others may lend support to this view (Brindle, 1989). For example, it is known that, statistically, women suffer from diagnosed mental illness far more than men do (Miles, 1981). Why is this? One view is that there actually *are* a greater number of mentally ill women than men, and this might be as a result of the sorts of lives they live in

111

what is still primarily a male-dominated society. Another view, however, is that there is a tendency for women to be *seen* as mentally ill more frequently than men. They, to a far greater degree than men, have to cope with certain role expectations, and acting outside of their role arouses disapproval. Behaviour that in men might be condoned, with the attitude 'boys will be boys', is not found acceptable in women. There are stories about women in the past being confined to mental hospitals, sometimes for many years, simply because they became pregnant out of wedlock.

Today, we like to think we are more enlightened, and it is to be hoped that this is true. But we are still constrained by all sorts of social rules and role expectations, and those whose behaviour does not conform may be seen as threatening by others. So is the anti-psychiatry movement right?

The 1983 Mental Health Act, despite its definitions, has not put an end to dispute. Section 1, for example, defines 'mental disorder' in terms of mental illness, but mental illness is not, itself, defined. The debate continues as to what, if anything, mental illness is.

The critics of psychiatry, however, while they have usefully drawn our attention to some of the uncertainties in diagnosis, ignore the following two points. First, they assume that diagnosis of all physical illness is value-free, whereas that of mental illness is not. The situation is far less clear-cut than this (Fulford, 1989). It may be that in each sphere there are some conditions which should not be 'medicalised'. This ties in with the second point, viz. that they ignore the difference between different *kinds* of mental illness. The basis of some is far more clearly understood than that of others. There is a danger, in dismissing mental illness as a myth, that people who really are very ill might be denied treatment. Despite the lack of clarity in the term, most people regard mental illness as a fact (Wilkes, 1988, p. 88).

Stigma

The diagnosis of mental illness is important for another reason, and that is because of the possibly serious consequences of such a diagnosis for the individual concerned. In our society there is still a stigma associated with mental illness, despite the fact that the Mental Health Acts 1959 and 1983 have attempted to improve the situation. It is a label that, once acquired, is very difficult to lose. As long as such social attitudes persist, there is a danger that health care professionals will also be affected by them, perhaps without realising it, and allow it to affect the quality of care that they give to patients. The horror stories that have emerged about standards in some mental hospitals in recent years seem to bear this out.

As Kathleen Wilkes points out, the problem may arise in part from the lack of mutual understanding between mentally ill and 'normal' people. Using the example of schizophrenia, she writes that it is 'difficult if not impossible to see the world through the mind of the schizophrenic, in terms of which the way he behaves seems, and might be shown to be, quite rational; and he for his part has temporarily, or perhaps even permanently, lost the ability to view the world as we do' (Wilkes, 1988, p. 90). Thus, mentally ill people seem 'different', and as a group may be discriminated against, like other groups we have discussed. But as Wilkes further points out: 'we must note that the mentally ill . . . are, since they belong to the same species, as like us as it is possible to be' (Wilkes, 1988, p. 98). She makes the interesting suggestion that it is in our capacity for mental illness that we are distinctive as a species. Our minds are so complex that they have greater potential to go wrong than those of other animals.

The point here is that mentally ill individuals are people, and thus are subject to the requirements of the principle of respect for persons.

The fact is, however, that in several respects mentally ill people *are* treated differently from others, and we must ask to what extent different treatment is justified. The first difference concerns the role of the nurse.

The power of the psychiatric nurse

Nurses are in a very unusual position with regard to mental illness. Section 5(4) of the 1983 Act provides that:

> If, in the case of a patient who is receiving treatment for mental disorder as an in-patient in a hospital, it appears to a nurse of the prescribed class:
> (a) that the patient is suffering from mental disorder to such a degree that it is necessary for his health or safety or for the protection of others for him to be immediately restrained from leaving the hospital; and
> (b) that it is not practicable to secure the immediate attendance of a practitioner for the purpose of furnishing a report . . . the nurse may record that fact in writing; and in that event the patient may be detained in the hospital for a period of six hours . . ..

As Clive Unsworth points out (Unsworth, 1987, p. 332), this section has serious implications for the relationship between nurse and patient, in that the nurse may be seen as a 'gaoler' rather than as a carer. The line between 'care' and 'control' is particularly difficult to draw in the treatment of mental illness but, says Unsworth, 'nurses are in . . . the front line of the mental health system in its character as an agency of social control' (Unsworth, 1987, p. 331). Anne Davis, though writing of the American system, speaks of the mental health nurse as a 'double agent': a regulatory agent for the state and a therapeutic agent for the patient (Davis, 1978).

This is one area of the law relating to nursing practice which sits very uneasily with the developing notion of advocacy. It may be true that the power is little used and that the nursing profession was not unanimous in supporting this change in its role (Unsworth, 1987, p. 332), but the fact that it is there displays the need for serious thought about what the role of the mental health nurse should be.

Also, a more general question arises here, about how, if at all, the detention of mentally ill people can be justified from a moral point of view.

The justification of detention

In addition to the nurse's limited power of detention, the 1983 Mental Health Act section 2(2) provides for an application for admission for assessment of a patient who (a) is suffering from mental disorder and (b) ought to be detained 'in the interests of his own health or safety or with a view to the protection of other persons'. While we must not overlook the fact that many people voluntarily seek treatment for mental illness, it is this power of compulsory detention that presents a moral dilemma.

Clause (b) claims to give us the justification for detention, and it falls into two parts: first, the interests of the patient, and second, the interests of others. Whether these justifications work has been very clearly examined by Richard Lindley (Lindley, 1978), and the discussion here will rely heavily on his arguments.

First, detaining someone for his own good is an instance of paternalism (cf Chapter 10). As we know, with 'normal' adults there is a presumption against paternalism. For example, we do not, as Lindley points out, think it right compulsorily to detain, 'in their own interests', people who smoke (Lindley, 1978, p. 31). In our society, we have a large measure of respect for the principle of autonomy, and if people want to take risks with their health we think that it is up to them. As a matter of fact we think that even though it may be, in one specific sense, against their interests to smoke, in another, wider, sense, it is in their own interests to be in charge of their own lives.

In the case of mentally ill people, we may suspect, especially if we have any sympathy with the anti-psychiatry movement, that they are detained, not in their own interests at all, but for the convenience of society. But let us assume that those with the power to detain genuinely believe that they are acting in the best interests of the patient. What is the difference, morally speaking, between the compulsory detention of a mentally ill person and that of a smoker?

According to Richard Lindley the difference lies in the fact that the smoker can weigh up the evidence for and against his course of action and take a decision, but in so far as a mentally ill person can justifiably be detained, it is because he has irrational beliefs, and thus is incapable of making rational decisions about his welfare.

> What is special about someone who has radically irrational
> beliefs of this kind is that he is likely, unwittingly, to get into all
> kinds of dangers. The person who believes he is indestructible
> might well walk into the middle of a busy road . . . he would not
> be moved by one's reasoning.
>
> (Lindley, 1978, p. 41)

If there *is* a justification for compulsory detention of mentally ill people in their own interests, this must surely be it. The mentally ill person, having irrational beliefs, has a diminished capacity for autonomy. There is a problem, of course, about what counts as an 'irrational' belief.

Some people take the view, for example, that potential suicides are inevitably irrational and ought to be prevented from taking their own lives. It is not difficult, however, to think of cases where, to a rational person, death might seem the most preferable of the available alternatives. So why the reluctance to respect the choice of the suicide? One answer is that the prevention of a suicide allows for the possibility of a change of mind and future exercise of autonomous choices, whereas death is the end of autonomy as of everything else. So interference can be justified, at least in some cases, for the sake of future autonomy. There is a problem, however, about how far we should take interference. Constant surveillance of a suicidal patient may be over-intrusive and counter-productive (Bydlon-Brown and Billman, 1988).

The second part of the justification for detention concerns the protection of others. As Lindley points out (Lindley, 1978, pp. 35–9), those mentally ill people who are detained on the grounds that they are dangerous fall into two categories: those who have already offended in some way, and those who are thought likely to offend. There is a particular problem with regard to the second group. Under normal circumstances, we do not think it justifiable to detain individuals who may harm others. Under the criminal law, persons are innocent until proven guilty. Why should the fact of mental illness justify making an exception to this? Lindley argues that it does not. We live in a society in which liberty is greatly prized, and in which the wrongful deprivation of that good is seen as a great wrong. Unless a relevant difference can be shown:

> it would seem arbitrary and unjust to treat mentally disturbed
> people as a special category. If we accept this preventive
> detention in the one case we should also do so in the other.
>
> (Lindley, 1978, p. 39)

This might lead us, for example, to lock up people 'who have committed no crimes, but, say, come from backgrounds which make it statistically likely that at some stage in their lives they will commit a serious crime' (Lindley, 1978, p. 36).

If we find this unacceptable we should think again about the preventive detention of mentally ill people.

Treatment

The right to refuse treatment in hospital

Many of the concerns expressed about the treatment of mental health have focused on the kinds of treatment involved and the ways in which they have been used. Electroconvulsive therapy (ECT) and psychosurgery, for example, have given rise to a great deal of controversy, sparked off by both academic debate and by novels such as Ken Kesey's *One Flew Over the Cuckoo's Nest* and Marge Piercy's *Woman on the Edge of Time*.

It is beyond the scope of our discussion to look at the details of the argument surrounding these treatments. If patients give informed consent to their use then the principle of autonomy suggests that it is up to them. Problems arise, however, when informed consent is lacking.

A question that has been much discussed in the USA in recent years is whether compulsorily detained patients have the right to refuse treatment. Does commitment necessarily involve losing one's rights to refuse? (Appelbaum, 1988). A number of courts in the USA have said that it does not; that a committed patient retains the right to have autonomous choices respected.

In the case of normal adults, as we have seen, the ethical doctrine of informed consent, which flows naturally from the principle of autonomy, holds that patients should be fully involved in decisions about their treatment, and to some extent this is enshrined in English law (*Sidaway vs. Board of Governors of the Bethlem Royal Hospital and the Maudsley Hospital*, 1985). To perform an operation, for example, on a normal adult against his will would count as a battery.

As regards mentally ill people, in the UK the 1983 Mental Health Act (section 3) explicitly provides for an application for admission for treatment. Further, section 63 makes it clear that, subject to certain exceptions, there is a power to treat without the consent of the patient. It reads:

> The consent of a patient shall not be required for any medical treatment given to him for the mental disorder from which he is suffering, not being treatment falling within section 57 or 58.

For example, according to section 57, psychosurgery requires consent and a second opinion.

It is clear from these sections that the Mental Health Act does recognise that some mentally ill patients are capable of giving or withholding consent. It is not the case that all patients are so ill that they are incapable of making an autonomous choice, though some are. These are said to lack 'competence'. To establish the criteria for determining competence is not a simple matter as we have seen elsewhere. What we need to consider, however, are those cases in which the patient is competent, but there exists the power to override his choice. Problem cases rarely concern those patients who consent to their treatment, as to whether they really were 'capable of understanding its nature, purpose and likely effects' (Mental Health Act, 1983, s.58 (3)(b)). Difficult issues arise when the patient refuses to give consent to a procedure which, in the eyes of the medical profession, is beneficial to his health.

The nurse has an important role to play here. Section 57, dealing with the conditions necessary for psychosurgery to be performed, provides a good example of this. The medical practitioner asking for a second opinion 'shall consult two other persons who have been professionally concerned with the patient's medical treatment, and of those persons one shall be a nurse'. As Unsworth comments, this is a 'novel incursion into territory previously dominated by the medical profession' (Unsworth, 1987, p. 325). It is one instance where the opportunity to speak for the patient, in order to protect his best interests, is written into the law. If there is room for the notion of nurse advocacy, it exists here (Bandman, 1978, p. 230).

Is there any justification, however, for refusing to respect the autonomy of mentally ill, but competent, patients in treatment decisions? For, as in the case of detention, they are being treated differently from other people.

One possible justification is that it is not just a question of distinguishing competent from incompetent people. As we noted when discussing detention, some patients, while they may satisfy criteria of competence, are irrational: their illness lessens their capacity for fully autonomous choices. So, by refusing to respect their choices, we may be fostering their autonomy rather than anything else (Sherlock, 1983, pp. 141–3). This argument parallels the argument for suicide prevention. In other words, restoring them to health is, in the long term, in the interests of a greater degree of autonomy.

This approach is not without its dangers. It is all too easy to call those who do not agree with our judgements irrational. Harry Lesser argues:

> Only if the phobia, or the depression or indecisiveness, is
> evidently preventing the patient from thinking clearly at all, or if
> it is combined with an inability to give any reason for his or her
> expressed preference, is one justified in regarding the
> preference . . . as irrational . . . and the patient – however irritating
> this may be to some doctors – should be considered 'rational
> until proved irrational'.

> (Lesser, 1983, p. 145)

How is this to be done? Hildegard Peplau suggests that the right to refuse treatment might follow participation in sessions designed to investigate conceptions of treatment and reasons for refusing (Peplau, 1978, p. 212).

For the nurse, who may be asked to give an opinion in these contexts, it is a question of examining whether the patient has been proved to be irrational, and whether the treatment will ultimately be in the interests of the patient's autonomy or not. While it is clear that without any compulsory treatment of mental illness some people would be worse off (Lindley, 1986, p. 150), any given instance requires justification.

Treatment in the community

The debate about refusal of treatment has recently taken a new twist with the move towards community care (DHSS, 1989). Among the factors that have encouraged this policy are modern drug treatments which make detention in hospital unnecessary (Lindley, 1986, pp. 157–8). Some patients who are discharged into the community, however, having earlier been detained for compulsory treatment, then refuse to continue their medications. Debate rages over the following issue, well put by David Brindle:

> If mentally ill people can be treated compulsorily in hospital, one side argues, why not also in the community now that more and more of them are living there? Because, retorts the other side, people deemed well enough to live in the community have the right to decide their own medication.
>
> (Brindle, 1990)

In the absence of the legal power to give compulsory treatment in the community, patients have the legal right to refuse. Some have argued, however, that it is in the interests of the patient to avoid compulsory readmission to hospital, and that therefore compulsory community treatment orders should be available (Brindle, 1990).

Morally, the same considerations apply as discussed above. If someone is capable of making a choice we should respect it. As Lesser says, only if there is clear evidence that the person is irrational are we justified in interfering to promote what we see as his good.

Confidentiality and the psychiatric patient

Another way in which the rights of mentally ill patients may be less well protected than those of others concerns confidentiality. In 1988 in the case of *W vs. Egdell and others* it was held that the duty of confidentiality that psychiatrists owe to patients detained under the Mental Health Act 1983 is less extensive than that owed to other patients, and that in some circumstances there is a duty of disclosure (Brahams, 1988, p. 1503).

In this case, a psychiatrist had disclosed facts about a patient's interest in making bombs, both to the medical director of the hospital where he was detained, and to the Home Office.

The extent of confidentiality owed to mentally ill people has been much discussed in the USA. In the well known *Tarasoff* case, a patient revealed to his therapist that he planned to kill his former girlfriend, Tatiana Tarasoff. He carried out the plan, and Tatiana's parents brought an action against the therapist for failure to warn. The court held that the question turned on whether a therapist should reasonably believe that his patient poses a threat to a third party. If the answer is yes, then the therapist must breach the confidence (Greenlaw, 1980, pp. 5 and 8).

In the later *Shaw* case, which involved the 'eternal triangle', a therapeutic team was treating husband, wife, and wife's lover. During the course of treatment, the wife left her husband for her lover, without revealing to her husband the lover's identity. The psychiatric nurse in the team, however, *did* convey this information, whereupon the husband shot the lover.

As Jane Greenlaw points out, one striking thing about the discussions of this case is that little or no mention has been made of the fact that it was a *nurse* who made the disclosure.

To say that, as a general rule, mentally ill patients are owed a less extensive duty of confidentiality is difficult to justify. The fact of mental illness alone is not a relevant difference sufficient to warrant breach of confidence. Nor, we would argue, is it sufficient that a patient is detained under the Mental Health Act. Many such patients pose no threat to others that could justify the disclosure of information about them. The difficult cases concern those who *are* thought to pose a threat to others. In such cases it seems to be a matter of weighing up the harm to the patient, in breaching confidentiality, against the possible harm the patient might do to others, and acting so as to achieve the least harm. But surely, it might be objected that the patient's interests must take priority? Some writers have argued, in reply, that to prevent a patient from harming others by a breach of confidentiality *is* in the patient's best interests – it is a kind of protection of the patient (Greenlaw, 1980, p. 5).

An important point is that patients who suffer from physical illness may also constitute a threat to the health of others. What we must observe, then, is that there are no grounds for saying that, as a group, mentally ill people have less right to confidentiality than do physically ill people.

What we can say is that there may be some cases when a breach is justified, but these will be very rare, and will generally be in order to protect other strong interests that are in conflict with the patient's interest in confidentiality (Chapter 1).

The nurse's breach of confidentiality in the *Shaw* case is difficult to condone. There is no apparent overriding justification in terms of the safety of others, and the fact that the wife and lover were receiving therapy does not excuse the passing on of this kind of information. People suffering from mental illness, like anyone else, have an interest in safeguarding their privacy.

The cases

Detention

❢ *As far as I was concerned she should have been allowed to go* ❣

A patient who was not legally bound to hospital one day left without informing anyone. As far as I was concerned she should have been allowed to go. However, the most senior member of staff sent me and another nurse to try to find the patient, suggesting that we look at the local shops, park and her home. Bearing in mind that we had no transport we had to walk about two miles to this patient's flat. Finding she was not there we began to walk back towards the hospital and discovered her walking by some shops. We then persuaded her to walk with us, not telling her that she would be going back to hospital. However, when we arrived at the police station (where she had previously worked) she refused to go any further. So, not knowing what to do, we asked a police officer to drive us back to the psychiatric hospital.

Commentary

This case shows that there may be very little practical difference between patients who are detained under a section of the Mental Health Act and those who are not. This patient was legally free to go, and yet her legal rights were not respected.

The legal question does not, of course, settle the moral question. From the moral point of view, we have seen that there are problems with the standard justifications of the compulsory detention of mentally ill people, but how would they apply in this case? There is no indication that this patient has been or is likely to be a danger to others. If she was, she would presumably be detained under a section of the Mental Health Act. So, the only conceivable justification for the action taken would be that it was in the interests of the patient. Following the arguments outlined above, whether such a justification works in a particular case would depend on whether the patient had irrational beliefs.

We are not given enough information to decide this question, but we do know that she was not thought to be suffering from such a degree of mental illness as to warrant compulsory detention under the Mental Health Act. Harry Lesser (1983) suggests that a patient should be assumed to be rational until proven irrational, but no attempt is made to persuade her, by argument, to consent to return to the hospital; no attempt is made to assess the extent to which this patient is capable of rational thought.

Instead, she is deceived. The patient is, in effect, coerced into returning with the nurses. As she is not a detained patient, she must have consented to be an in-patient originally. Thus, her capacity to give genuine consent was not disputed with regard to that decision. It is when exercise of choice disagrees with that of the health care professionals that problems arise. For mentally ill people, their 'choice' in effect may be between consent to admission, or compulsory admission, but not between admission and no admission at all.

It is difficult to believe that the situation of mentally ill people as a whole will improve while it is thought acceptable by health care professionals to disregard their legal rights, and to presume that they are irrational until proven otherwise, rather than the other way round.

Punishment or treatment?

❝ I have had to argue with doctors who insist on medicating or secluding a patient unlawfully ❞

I work on a psychiatric unit. Several times I have had to argue with doctors who insist on medicating or secluding a patient unlawfully (eg. using seclusion as a punishment). While I find that to be an easy question (I am a patient advocate) I find going against another nurse's judgment to be more problematic. I have often heard nurses speak of 'medicating (with tranquillisers) early' when we are short-staffed or overcrowded.

The most difficult problem comes when a nurse, especially a nurse I respect, wants to seclude a patient because she is angry – for example, with a patient who uses racial slurs. When they call for help I help them, but should I help when I know they are wrong?

Commentary

The nurse in this case is clear, first, that it is wrong to treat patients in the ways described. The care setting is not intended for punishment.

The boundary between 'care' and 'control', however, may become blurred, and 'control' can easily slip into punishment. Of course, some patients are compulsorily detained in mental hospitals because they have committed the sorts of deeds that would, but for their illness, have justified imprisonment. This fact does not justify, however, overlooking the fact that the purposes of the two kinds of institution are fundamentally different.

The fact of detention, together with the move towards the 'nurse as gaoler' role, may lead to a situation in which nurses are more likely to see their role as a custodial one. This would not fit well alongside the Code of Conduct. But whether or not nurses see themselves in this light, the fact is that there is an unequal power relationship betwen nurses and their patients which is more marked in the mental health setting, where a large proportion of those receiving treatment may not be free to leave.

The fact that some patients will be unrewarding to care for is a fact of life. It may well be offensive for a nurse to hear patients expressing racist views, especially if they are directed against the nurse herself. However, to punish a patient for that by the use of methods intended for other purposes, is to take unfair advantage of the inequality in power that already exists.

The temptation to medicate early is understandable. It may appear that, if the medication has to be given anyway, then why not give it a little earlier, to make life easier for the staff? However, this view is wrong in that it encourages the view that medication may be administered for the benefit of the nurses, rather than for the benefit of the patients. If the problem results from serious staffing shortages, the Code of Conduct urges that attention should be drawn to this fact (UKCC, 1984). To speak in this way might be thought idealistic – there always will be resource problems, it might be claimed. The point is, however, that it is undesirable for nurses to adopt the frame of mind that nothing can be done. The passive acceptance of unsatisfactory circumstances can have harmful consequences both for the morale of nurses and for the welfare of patients. The UKCC Advisory Document, *Exercising Accountability*, says that it is essential that the profession 'achieve high standards rather than . . . simply accept minimum standards' (UKCC, 1989, p. 7). This is particularly important in the context of mental health.

The final point in this case concerns the nurse's point about being a patient advocate. She writes that she has no problem about arguing with doctors, but where other nurses are concerned, it is a different story. What she says demonstrates some of the unclarities and difficulties in the notion of advocacy (Chapter 2). The author appears to see it as involving conflict with other professionals, primarily doctors, but wants to avoid conflict with her peers. And yet, if she is to speak for patients this must involve protecting them from abuse by other nurses as well as from doctors. The case illustrates that it may be more profitable to concentrate on Clause 1 of the Code of Conduct than on the concept of advocacy.

Consent to treatment I

❝ *The patient was held down . . . I was instructed to give her an injection to sedate her* ❞

During my experience on a psychiatric ward, one of our day-patients was slightly more aggressive than usual. Because of this, she disturbed the psychotherapy group which was going on. Her parents were telephoned to collect her. When they arrived, however, they decided that their daughter's behaviour was disgusting and demanded that some sort of sedative should be given despite the protests of the patient and the charge nurse.

Unfortunately the consultant agreed with the parents (as did all the other medical staff), so the patient was held down on a bed in a side ward and I was instructed to give her an injection to sedate her. I was distressed at the situation; the patient clearly gave her view and it was against her will. The patient was not on any Mental Health Act Section. However I gave the drug because it was prescribed by the consultant, and the staff nurse insisted that I should give it because I was the only woman on that particular shift.

Commentary

The nurse points out that the action proposed cannot be justified under the Mental Health Act. Also, it morally violates the principle of informed consent. There is no suggestion that the patient is not competent to consent. It is difficult to find anything in favour, morally speaking, of the forced medication.

We are not given details as to the ways in which the behaviour of this patient was found to be 'disgusting', but we have to remember that to subject the body of another human being to force may also be viewed as disgusting. It is not a course of action that we would find acceptable in the normal course of events. The incident shows how different standards are operated for those recognised as mentally ill, such that, in the case before us, even the parents find it easier to accept the violation of their daughter's rights than her behaviour.

There is no suggestion that she is dangerous to others, so the medication cannot be justified as an emergency measure for protection purposes. Nor does it seem to have been done in the patient's own interests, but rather for the convenience of others.

One interesting feature of the incident is that all the medical staff agree that to give the injection is correct, while the nurses do not. And yet, it is a nurse who has to carry out the order, against her will. If she were to disobey, she might well be disciplined.

The only way, however, to protect mentally ill people from invasions of their legal rights and from being the victims of moral wrongs, is for individuals to refuse to participate in or condone them.

Consent to treatment II

> ❮ The nurse has to 'cover' for the doctor ❯

A doctor on my ward was in the habit of changing patients' medications without telling the patient. For example, he would increase or decrease the dosage; add to or delete medicines. One particular patient, suffering from paranoia, already had trust problems and a tendency to non-compliance. When she did not receive the 'right' number, or the usual colour, of pills, this encouraged further lack of trust in the nurse–doctor 'system'. The nurse has to 'cover' for the doctor in order to gain compliance and trust. In my opinion, each member of the health care team must be responsible and accountable to tie up loose ends, instead of leaving unfinished business and its consequences for the nurse to deal with.

Commentary

This case is an expression of disapproval at the ways in which nurses have to deal with problems that are caused or made worse by other members of. the team. This is a general point, but the specific example is particularly relevant to the case of mentally ill people.

The doctor on this psychiatric ward clearly does not trouble to discuss treatment with the patients. And yet, as Lindley points out, this is not asking for very much. He writes: 'A small step towards respecting autonomy would be for doctors, as a general rule, to explain to patients what the different treatment options might be' (Lindley, 1986, pp. 161–2). The case description shows that omitting to do this is unacceptable from the point of view of the principle of autonomy, and that it is actually bad for patients' health. In other words, there are also consequentialist grounds for respecting autonomy. If patients are treated with respect they are more likely to comply, with better results for their own health. Unfortunately, as we have seen, in the psychiatric setting it is more likely than it is elsewhere that the opinions of patients will be disregarded.

Should the nurse confront this doctor? The UKCC, in *Exercising Accountability*, says that when a nurse feels that sufficient information has not been given 'it is for her to state this opinion and seek to have the situation remedied' (UKCC, 1989, p. 10). This might take considerable courage, but could be done in this case in the form of asking him to have a word with this particular patient about her medication. Nurses are accountable for themselves but not for other members of the health care team, as the writer points out.

Conclusion

We have seen that there is a danger that mentally ill people may be treated in ways that cannot be justified simply on the grounds of mental illness alone. The nurse, however, in this context perhaps even more than in others, has it in her power to make a real difference to their standards of care, and to monitor the moral acceptability of their treatment.

References

Appelbaum, P. S. (1988) 'The right to refuse treatment with antipsychotic medications: retrospect and prospect', *American Journal of Psychiatry*, vol. 145, pp. 413–19.

Bandman, E. L. (1978) 'The right of the mentally ill to refuse treatment', in E. L. Bandman and B. Bandman (eds), *Bioethics and Human Rights: A Reader for Health Professionals*, pp. 224–32 (Boston: Little, Brown & Co.).

Bloch, S. (1984) 'The political misuse of psychiatry in the Soviet Union', in S. Bloch and P. Chodoff, (eds) *Psychiatric Ethics* (Oxford: Oxford University Press).

Brahams, D. (1988) 'A psychiatrist's duty of confidentiality', *The Lancet*, 24/31 December, pp. 1503–4.

Brindle, D. (1989) 'Racial stereotyping blamed for discrepancies in mental detention', *Guardian*, 17 April.

Brindle, D. (1990) 'Keep taking the tablets', *Guardian*, 3 Jan.

Bydlon-Brown, B. and Billman, R. R. (1988) 'At risk for suicide . . . ', *American Journal of Nursing*, vol. 88, pp. 1358–62.

Davis, A. J. (1978) 'The ethics of behavior control: the nurse as double agent', *Issues in Mental Health Nursing*, vol. 1, pp. 2–16.

Department of Health and Social Security (DHSS) (1989) *Caring for People: Community Care in the Next Decade and Beyond* (London: HMSO).

Fulford, K. W. M. (1989) *Moral Theory and Medical Practice* (Cambridge: CUP).

Greenlaw, J. (1980) 'Confidentiality – the psychotherapist's nemesis', *Nursing Law and Ethics*, vol. 1, pp. 5, 8.

Lesser, H. (1983) 'Consent, competency and ECT: a philosopher's comment', *Journal of Medical Ethics*, vol. 9, pp. 144–5.

Lindley, R. (1978) 'Social Philosophy', in R. Lindley *et al*, *What Philosophy Does* (London: Open Books).

Lindley, R. (1986) *Autonomy* (Houndmills: Macmillan).

Mental Health Acts 1959 and 1983.

Miles, A. (1981) *The Mentally Ill in Contemporary Society* (Oxford: Martin Robertson).

Peplau, H. (1978) 'The right to change behavior: rights of the mentally ill', in E. L. Bandman, and B. Bandman (eds) *Bioethics and Human Rights: A Reader for Health Professionals*, pp. 207–12 (Boston: Little, Brown & Co.).

Sherlock, R. (1983) 'Consent, competency and ECT: some critical suggestions', *Journal of Medical Ethics*, vol. 9, pp. 141–3.

Sidaway vs Board of Governors of the Bethlem Royal Hospital and the Maudsley Hospital (1985).

Szasz, T. S. (1962) *The Myth of Mental Illness* (London: Harper & Row).

United Kingdom Central Council for Nursing, Midwifery and Health Visiting (1984) *Code of Professional Conduct for the Nurse, Midwife and Health Visitor*, 2nd ed. (London: UKCC).

United Kingdom Central Council for Nursing, Midwifery and Health Visiting (1989) *Exercising Accountability: A Framework to Assist Nurses, Midwives and Health Visitors to Consider Ethical Aspects of Professional Practice* (London: UKCC).

Unsworth, C. (1987) *The Politics of Mental Health Legislation* (Oxford: Clarendon Press).

Wilkes, K. V. (1988) *Real People: Personal Identity Without Thought Experiments* (Oxford: Clarendon Press).

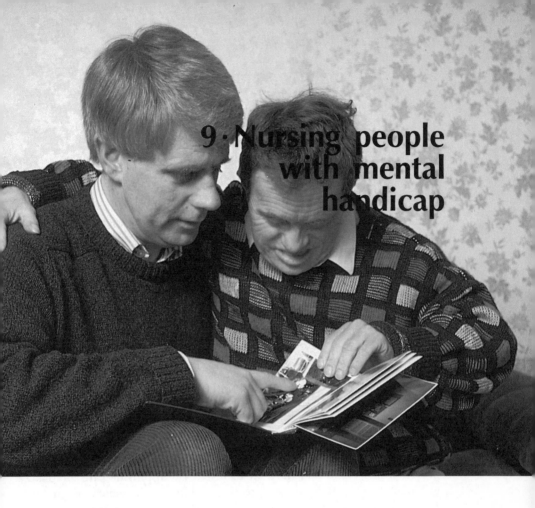

9 · Nursing people with mental handicap

Introduction

Nursing in the field of mental handicap is presently in the process of great change. The reasons for the changes are many, but include the shift towards community-based care resulting first, from the 1971 White Paper, 'Better Services for the Mentally Handicapped' and later from the adoption of the philosophy of normalisation. This has meant a greater involvement of the social services and other agencies outside of traditional health care, in the continuing care of clients.

Advancing medical technology and, in particular, genetic engineering and pre-natal screening have forced society to examine its values in relation to people with a mental handicap. Increasing awareness of the needs of mentally handicapped individuals, with the advent of the 1981 Education Act, as well as a general increase in demand for the rights of minority groups to be recognised, have all led to a sharpening of public interest in this area of health care.

Social discrimination and isolation

Historically, the subject of mental handicap has always been value-laden, and it is important to recognise this before trying to analyse and understand today's issues. In ancient Greece, Aristotle did not view defective infants as capable of human endeavour; the Romans and Spartans had laws under which the handicapped could be exterminated in infancy; religious leaders such as Martin Luther and John Calvin believed that such individuals were possessed by the devil and should be executed. In medieval Europe, the handicapped were, at best, tolerated as jesters or freaks, and at worst were feared as creatures of Satan and dealt with accordingly. In the 17th century, confinement and isolation with criminals, the poor and the insane began and this became the accepted pattern of care provision.

Throughout the 18th and 19th centuries asylums and institutions for mentally ill and handicapped people became more widespread. With the advent of the eugenics movement, propaganda about the mentally handicapped flourished and the condition was rapidly viewed as resulting from a life of degeneration which, unless contained, would ultimately result in social and financial hardships for the remainder of society. This resulted in even more stringent isolation and restrictive laws in relation to marriage, propagation and property (de Leon Siantz, 1979, pp. 57–67).

The term mental handicap has, to a large extent, been viewed more as a social status than as a medical problem, and this has affected the provision of services and the staff themselves who provide care for this group of people. Reports of appalling conditions, in which mentally handicapped people were forced to live, were common news items in the sixties and seventies. There were accounts of ill-treatment on both sides of the Atlantic, for example Willowbrooks (Rivera, 1972) and Ely (DHSS, 1969).

These enquiries certainly brought to light the disturbing facts that had been hidden and ignored over the years, and forced society to question how we ought to treat individuals with mental impairment. Whether or not we have learned to value mentally handicapped people more than we did in the past is still the subject of much debate and is an important issue especially in light of the Government's White Paper for Community Care (DHSS, 1989) which discusses the care of people in the community in the future.

Valuing an individual requires more than discharging them from institutional care. It involves seeking his opinion about issues that affect his day-to-day life. This is a crucial aspect of respecting individuals as persons as to disregard someone's wishes is to treat him as something less than a person (*see*, also, the discussion on mental illness in chapter 8).

Paternalism

Paternalism is commonly agreed to be the overriding of an individual's autonomy, for the purpose of acting in his best interests. The justification for this is that the individual is judged to be incapable of making a rational choice, as we have already seen in the case of a young child.

In other words, paternalism is closely associated with the principles beneficence and non-maleficence, as its justification rests on the premise that one ought to promote the welfare of other individuals (beneficence), or at least prevent harm befalling them (non-maleficence) if we suspect that their autonomous choices are based on impaired thinking or misinformation which may lead to the suffering of unnecessary harms. The rationale for paternalism is always the desire to safeguard an individual's best interest.

Philosphers often distinguish between two forms of paternalism, strong and weak. Strong paternalism is generally agreed to be the limiting or denial of a person's freedom of choice, even when that person's choices are made on an informed and voluntary basis. The concept of weak paternalism is, however, less clear cut and frequently more readily accepted. Joel Feinberg distinguishes weak paternalism as 'the right to prevent self-regarding conduct only when it is substantially nonvoluntary or when temporary intervention is necessary to establish whether it is voluntary or not' (Feinberg, 1973, p. 63).

Proponents of paternalism often argue that we all accept weak paternalism as part of our everyday lives as for instance in the case of laws restricting speed or the amount of alcohol that drivers are permitted to drink. But whether or not these constitute examples of weak paternalism is open to debate.

It could be argued that the intention of such regulations in our lives is primarily the protection of others rather than the individual directly affected. If this is the case then such regulations are based on the *harm* principle and not on paternalism (Tadd, 1989, p. 33).

One serious problem with paternalism is that any choice that is perceived to be unconventional is likely to be overruled especially if a result of the choice may be harmful to the individual. It is of course always the interventionist's perception of harm which rules, especially if the choice made is likely to be at odds with the choice that the majority of people would make in similar circumstances. In such situations, this in itself may be cited as evidence that paternalistic intervention is necessary, on the grounds that such an idosyncratic choice can only be the result of an irrational mind.

All too often mentally handicapped people are automatically assumed to be incapable of making their own decisions and choices. In other words, their capacity for autonomous decision-making is thought to be impaired and, while this may be acceptable in cases where the individual is profoundly handicapped, it is not necessarily the case with the mildly handicapped individual. Quite recently, national television reported a young woman with Down's syndrome as having passed her driving test, an activity which requires making many rational decisions. (It is worth remembering that the majority of mentally handicapped people are classified as being either moderately or mildly handicapped.)

Rights

Today, the language of rights is so commonplace that it is easy to forget that, historically, the concept of rights is relatively new. A popular assumption is that all members of mankind ought to possess equal human rights.

A right is defined by the Oxford English Dictionary as 'a justified claim to have or receive something, or to act in a certain way' and they are often classified as being either positive or negative. Feinberg defines these as follows, 'a positive right is a right to other persons' positive actions; a negative right is a right to other persons' forbearances or omissions' (Feinberg, 1973, p. 38).

If 'A' claims a right to health care or education then he is claiming a positive right as an obligation is placed on others to provide a service. For this reason positive rights are also referred to as welfare rights. The difficulty of course lies in determining where or on whom this obligation can rightfully be placed. For example, the right to education demands that 'B' and 'C' are prepared to become teachers. As 'B' and 'C' also have rights to embark on a career of their own choosing, it is difficult to see how 'As' claim can be secured if no-one is prepared to enter the teaching profession.

Negative rights are often referred to as liberty or option rights as the only obligation on others is to refrain from interfering when the right holder exercises his claim. An often cited example of such a right is the right to free speech.

One important aspect of rights theory is that rights are equal and must be universally applied. Further, most supporters of rights theory would agree that rights are not absolute. For example, many people would accept that all people have an equal right to life or at least a right not to be killed. In some circumstances, however, this right may be justifiably overridden. In exercising the right to protect his life an individual may be left with no alternative but to end the life of an attacker in the cause of self-defence.

Another difficulty with rights theory is that rights are competitive. When one person claims a right he is typically claiming them against someone else who may also believe that his rights are being overruled, and there are no clear mechanisms for determining whose claims should prevail or whose rights have priority (Tadd and Chadwick, 1989, p. 585).

In the case of legal rights then, we would look to legal principles and, if necessary, to the courts to adjudicate. In the case of moral rights, however, there is frequently no agreement about the primacy of particular moral principles and therefore there is significant scope for conflicts which may be both difficult and painful to resolve (Tadd and Chadwick, 1989, p. 585).

Rights theory is frequently appealed to in protecting the interests of minority groups, and mentally handicapped people may be seen as a minority group.

Sexuality

One aspect of the mentally handicapped individual's life which is perpetually prone to intrusion and external interference is that of sexuality. To some extent this has been made worse over recent months by high court rulings which have enabled mentally handicapped women to be sterilised without their consent, and it may be useful to explore the grounds on which these decisions were made.

In 1987, the House of Lords ruled that Jeanette, a 17-year-old girl with an approximate mental age of five, should be sterilised 'in her own interests'. Lord Dillon one of the Law Lords was quoted as saying, 'the consequences of her becoming pregnant were frightening' (Re B, 1987). For the judges, the possible pain and emotional trauma of childbirth were deemed sufficient justification to interfere with Jeanette's right to parenthood. By portraying a potential pregnancy as a possible cause of pain, suffering or even death and then introducing the principle of non-maleficence, that is the duty to prevent possible harm, sterilisation was seen as being in the individual's best interest.

While no-one would want to deny that occasionally women do die as a result of either pregnancy or childbirth, it is equally true that people can also die having a general anaesthetic for relatively minor surgery such as sterilisation. Likewise, while labour and the process of childbirth is not without pain, neither is the postoperative period following even minor surgery. As we have no guarantee that Jeanette would become pregnant it would seem to be just as logical to remove her appendix, her gallbladder and indeed her molars just in case they too become a source of pain that she would not understand.

As already mentioned, it is in no way certain that Jeanette would ever become pregnant, let alone experience an unduly painful labour and, at the age of 17 years, it seems a little premature to say that the complexities of contraception will forever remain beyond her capabilities. Such grounds for advocating sterilisation as being in her best interests appear unconvincing.

An alternative reason put forward as a justification for sterilisation of the mentally handicapped without consent, is that a mentally handicapped woman is unlikely to make a 'good' parent. However, if incompetence in parenting is to be used as a justification for denying the right to reproduce, then, as Wolfensburger points out, ' . . . it should be applied to the retarded and the non-retarded alike, and many bright, well educated persons are unfit parents' (Wolfensburger, cited in Craft, 1983).

It seems reasonable that ' . . . if a right to parenthood exists, then a valid reason for overriding that right may be on the grounds that an individual would unduly neglect the child, or cause injury to it' (Tadd, 1989, p. 16).

Using such arguments, it is easy to see that there are a large number of people who may legitimately be denied the right to parent a child, for example, known child abusers, drug addicts, psychopaths or, possibly, even heavy smokers or compulsive gamblers.

Without the formulation of specific criteria to determine an individual's 'fitness to parent', it is unjust to use such incompetence as grounds for compulsory sterilisation of the mentally handicapped alone.

Despite the direction that Jeanette's case should not be regarded as a precedent, Mr Justice Baker in a second case in 1988, ruled that a 35-year-old mentally handicapped woman should be sterilised, despite the fact that she was unable to give consent for the operation (*F vs. West Berkshire HA, 1988*). The woman's mother had sought the ruling as her daugher, whom it is said had a mental age of four years, had formed a sexual relationship with a male patient who resided in the same institution.

What is particularly disturbing about this judgement is that apparently 'F' was considered competent with regard to consenting to a sexual relationship but not, however, competent to give consent for surgery and, as Carsons points out, 'If there is no need to protect 'F' against exploitation and infectious disease, is there really a need to protect her against pregnancy?' (Carsons, 1989, pp. 690–1).

In upholding the decision to allow the sterilisation of 'F', the House of Lords ruled that the standard to be applied in determining what was in an individual's best interest should be the same as that used in 1987 in *Bolam vs. Friern Hospital Management Committee.*

However, that particular standard was used to determine medical negligence, and not what might or might not be in an individual's best interests. Therefore, it can be argued that it is not wholly appropriate.

In criticising this judgement, Carsons draws an analogy between the law relating to children, and the test that is used in deciding best interests. In such cases, decisions are based on an objective inquiry, which emphasises that the interests of the child are more important than those of the parents or indeed the administrative convenience of a public body. Decisions are not based on the opinion of one group of professionals, which is the test for negligence (Carsons, 1989, p. 13).

It is particularly disturbing that, as a number of similar cases are waiting to be heard, the law has seemingly reinforced the power of both medical and parental paternalism over the lives of mentally handicapped people. Sterilisation now appears to be viewed as the first choice in an array of treatments, rather than as a last resort. Nurses need to consider their opinions carefully, as their necessary involvement in such cases is obvious and, as we are all too well aware, legal sanction in no way determines the moral correctness of an action.

Many nurses caring for mentally handicapped people have described incidents when the sexual rights of men and women had been overruled. For example, one nurse who was interviewed described how a 25-year-old woman was prescribed and given depot injections as a contraceptive measure. The woman herself was given no explanation of the side-effects of this treatment over the long-term or indeed any choice as to her preferred method of contraception. The parents' wishes were the only ones considered and it was their decision upon which the medical staff acted.

Another nurse discussed how a 25-year-old resident was discouraged from forming a relationship with a 55-year-old mildly retarded man who was living in the community. When the staff's attempts to discourage the relationship failed, the man was refused permission to visit his girlfriend and the young woman was forcibly physically examined after she had been away from the hospital premises.

These cases and the ones which we will now discuss highlight the injustices and discriminatory practices sometimes applied in nursing mentally handicapped people.

The cases

Informed consent

❛ *There was nothing in his records to show that Bill had given his consent* ❜

While working on a ward for moderately handicapped male residents, I was allocated to care for Bill, a 27-year-old man. I was curious to know his history as he had very apparent secondary sexual characteristics of an obviously feminine nature, namely silky smooth skin and quite large breasts. This was a source of amusement to some of the other residents and I felt sympathy towards Bill whenever he was teased by his peers.

On reading his case notes it became clear that he had first been treated with a libido suppressing drug after being caught exposing himself to an elderly lady in a public park. Although not charged with any offence, he was returned by the police to the hospital.

For the last three years this young man had been given a daily dose of a libido-reducing drug resulting in his body taking on the described appearance.

There was nothing in his records to show that Bill had given his consent, let alone had the side-effects of his treatment explained and on checking with the charge nurse, I was told that Bill had never complained about his treatment.

Commentary

Obviously the community, and particularly those members that are most vulnerable, must be protected from sexual abuse, but at the same time it is essential to guard against hysterical overreaction. A normal man found guilty of a similar crime would have been fined or placed on a probation order for a first offence, but whatever his punishment, it would certainly have been for a determinate period.

By way of contrast, this young man's treatment appears severe and unremitting. A utilitarian may wish to argue that as Bill himself appeared happy with the treatment, then there was no dilemma as everyone's interests seem to be served. Despite the fact that the treatment had been effective in that he no longer exposed himself and his family are very happy with the 'therapy' as they are spared any embarrassment when he visits them for holidays, one needs to ask whether such treatment would have been adopted had the 'offender' been anything other than mentally handicapped. Whether chemical castration is an appropriate solution is doubtful, especially before any alternatives have been tried.

The sadness of this case is reflected in the fact that there must be many Bills up and down the country, subjected to similar forms of treatment. It appears that the cost to the individual is very low on the list of priorities when treatments are chosen, the most important criterion being how efficiently the problem behaviour is eradicated. The notion of consent, not to mention informed consent, is apparently ignored or is thought to be inappropriate.

Acting paternalistically

❛ The nurse attempted to force feed her ❜

I was working on a mixed ward for more able mentally handicapped residents. Mary was 54 years of age and approximately two stone overweight according to her height–weight ratio. She enjoyed her food and had no medical problems. However, the ward sister decided that she should be placed on a reducing diet. Mary was generally well behaved and was capable of going into town on her own, dressing herself and maintaining her own hygiene. However, after a few days of being on her diet, she was caught stealing food from other residents and on more than one occasion, taking food from the rubbish bins.

On one particular Friday, it was fish on the menu. All of the other residents had fried fish and chips, but Mary was given boiled cod. She expressed her dislike of the food and said she did not want to eat it. One of the qualified staff forced her back into her seat and repeatedly shouted at her saying, 'You will eat this food'. When Mary still refused, the nurse attempted to force feed her.

Mary became very distressed over the incident, and gradually appeared withdrawn and depressed. I spoke to the ward sister, saying that I felt it was unkind, that Mary should have some choice in the matter of her diet especially as she was a voluntary resident, and that force feeding isn't even allowed in prison.

The sister brushed aside my complaints saying, 'It will be good for Mary to lose weight and anyway we can't let her get the better of us can we?'. The sister's attitude was made much worse by the fact that she herself was at least three stones overweight.

I think it is cruel and disrespectful to treat people in this way, particularly as Mary was punished for stealing food.

Commentary

This sad story highlights a number of issues that are particularly relevant to nurses working in the field of mental handicap. One of these is that of paternalism which we have already discussed in general terms.

Considering Mary's case, it is necessary to ask if the sister's paternalistic actions were justified? Presumably she felt that Mary's health was compromised by her being overweight. Mary's own preference was to eat the food she enjoyed, despite the fact that it was high in calories. This, of course, is exactly the way that many people of normal intelligence choose to live. After all, knowing the calorific value of certain foods is no guarantee that they will not be eaten, even by individuals who have chosen to lose weight, as those of us who have tried to diet and failed, know all too well.

Leaving aside for the moment the questionable manner in which Mary was treated, is it justifiable for nurses to make these kinds of decisions for informal patients? Let us imagine that, instead of being generally medically fit, Mary had suffered a heart attack and had high blood pressure which could precipitate further illness at any time. It could then be argued that the sister had an overriding duty of care, to restrict

Mary's food intake and, if necessary, to do so against her wishes, should Mary refuse to comply.

Most reasonable people would no doubt agree that when a life-threatening situation exists and the individual concerned is not responding rationally to the danger, then paternalistic intervention is justifiable. However, Mary's situation is hardly life threatening and there is a large proportion of the population who take the view that today's pleasure is worth the risk of tomorrow's ill-health, or put another way, they would rather live 'a short life but a good one'.

Mary may, therefore, be acting rationally in wanting to eat the fried fish, especially when one considers the bleakness of institutional life, in which, for some residents, the only highlights of the day are mealtimes. It may be that the ward sister and the nurses involved in this scenario feel that because they are more intelligent than Mary, this alone justifies them making decisions on her behalf. If this is so, then it is a dangerous assumption for, as Wikler (1979, pp. 377–92) argues, if people of normal intelligence can make decisions for mildly handicapped individuals, then it is logical that gifted persons should make decisions for those of us who are of normal intelligence.

Bearing in mind the sister's obesity, I wonder how she would respond if after choosing a delicious but high calorie meal, a doctor or a dietician stepped forward and took her plate saying 'You can't eat that, have a salad instead!'. It needs to be emphasised that a cardinal rule in ethical deliberation is that the principles must be universally applied.

Wikler himself puts up an argument against this notion of superiority of intellect, when he suggests that perhaps what is necessary is a threshold level of intelligence above which it is possible to make one's own decisions. Superiority above that level is merely a bonus. Those who accept that explanation must accept that the onus is on them to determine scientifically what the necessary level of intellect is, and that is particularly difficult.

Nurses, especially those involved in caring for the moderately or mildly handicapped must exercise restraint over the sometimes natural tendency to make decisions blithely on behalf of their clients. If they fail to do this, then they can be rightly accused of treating such individuals as something less than persons.

Another important point to make in this case concerns the nature of paternalism. In our definition, we stated that paternalism involved overriding an individual's autonomy in his own best interests. In other words, the individual should benefit from the intervention and not be worse off.

In Mary's case, however, the decision to restrict her food intake resulted in Mary rummaging through waste bins for extra food. It is difficult to imagine how Mary can benefit from this state of affairs. Indeed, it is damaging to her as a person, for it is undignified and constitutes a serious risk to Mary's health.

The whole unpleasant situation is made worse by the manner in which the staff chose to pursue their goals, for example shouting and forcing Mary to eat food which she did not like, not to mention the student's suggestion that the sister saw herself in competition with Mary. No aspect of the staff's behaviour reflects the standard expected of a professional in a caring role.

Infringing personal freedom

❛ The charge nurse wasn't very pleased with my criticism and told me that I would be in trouble ❜

While gaining experience on a ward for more able residents, I spent a great deal of my time with Robert, a 42-year-old man. From time to time he liked to write letters to his sister, who was his only relative. Robert made a great play of buying note paper and envelopes and would then ask for help in spelling the odd word. His letters were really simple notes which contained nothing of an offensive nature.

After writing, he would buy a stamp from the hospital shop and ask one of the staff to post the letter for him on their way home. The first occasion I helped Robert to write his letter, he asked me to post it. I readily agreed and placed the letter in my pocket. The charge nurse who was in the ward at the time called me into the office. He asked for the letter and to my horror when I passed it to him, he tore it up and dropped it into the waste bin, saying that we were not to post any of Robert's scribblings to his sister.

I asked why, and he said that the sister did not want any contact with her brother. Politely I tried to explain that I disagreed with this action as it was an offence to tamper with anyone's mail and if the sister did not want any contact then she could destroy the letters.

The charge nurse wasn't very pleased with my criticism and told me that I would be in trouble if he caught me posting letters for Robert.

I resolved there and then to help Robert with his letters when the charge nurse was off-duty and to show him how to post them for himself so that he would not have to rely on the staff. Later, I asked the staff nurse what she thought of the charge nurse's actions but she could see nothing wrong as Robert was happy, his sister was happy and the staff were happy.

Commentary

Here we find a student nurse being reprimanded and threatened for trying to defend a resident's rights to send a letter. Correctly, she points out that if the person receiving the letter does not wish to read it, then she is the one who should destroy it. After all, one has no control over what drops through one's letter box, only over what one reads.

No doubt Robert's sister had complained to staff in the past and, instead of the staff encouraging her to tell her brother that she does not wish to receive any communication from him, the staff have opted for a quiet life and chosen to destroy the letters. The staff nurse does not appear to realise that anything unethical is taking place when she says that in adopting these actions everyone is happy.

This highlights why it is important for nurses to challenge from time to time, not only their own thinking, but also that of others. What is actually happening in this situation, is that Robert's freedom to communicate is being jeopardised and that of course can be the first step on what could become a slippery slope.

Imagine if the local Member of Parliament said that he did not wish to receive letters from his constituents and persuaded someone to intercept them before they arrived at his office. We would certainly wish to claim that our right to be represented was being severely impaired and some of us might take action to ensure that the honourable, or in this case dishonourable, member was suitably punished. Alternatively, consider what the staff might do if a resident said that he wanted to write a letter of complaint about them. It is difficult to believe that such a letter would not be destroyed.

The student correctly recognises that to enable Robert to exercise his freedom to communicate adequately, he needs to be taught how to post his letters, thereby decreasing his dependence on the staff. In fact, she seems to have recognised what the charge nurse and staff nurse have failed to realise and that is, that when charged with the responsibility for caring for dependent individuals, regardless of the nature of the dependence, the nurse must exercise extreme ethical caution, as the potential for abuse is great.

What is particularly distressing in this case is the deceit that has obviously taken place over time. No doubt Robert has carefully written his notes and handed them over to the staff in the belief that they would be posted, only for them to be secretly destroyed. Again, we seem to have a situation where an individual is treated very differently from the way in which the majority would expect to be treated, on the sole basis that his intelligence is impaired. As such grounds do not constitute a morally relevant difference, then we can conclude that such treatment is unjust.

Conclusion

Normally, we would expect that those suffering from disabilities of any nature, would be deserving of extra protection, particularly from individuals charged with the responsibility of giving care and yet, it appears that this is not always so. Indeed, these cases have highlighted how some of the staff themselves appear to have become immune to the needs of their charges.

With today's philosophy of closing institutions and moving people who are mentally handicapped out into the community, it is vital that these vulnerable members of our society, are treated not only with compassion, but also that they are afforded protection against social injustice and inhuman treatment.

References

Carsons, D. (1989) 'Sterilisation: Whose Body Is It Anyway?', *Health Service Journal*, Jan 5, p. 13.

Carsons, D. (1989) 'Why the Law Lords Said Yes To Sterilisation', *Health Service Journal*, Jun 8, pp. 690–1.

de Leon Siantz, M. L. (1979) 'Human Values In Determining The Fate Of Persons With Mental Retardation', *Nursing Clinics of North America*, vol. 14, no. 1, pp. 57–67.

DHSS (1969) *Report of the Committee of Inquiry Into Allegations of Ill-treatment of Patients and Other Irregularities at Ely Hospital Cardiff* (London: HMSO; Cmnd 3975).

DHSS (1989) *Caring For People: Community Care in The Next Decade and Beyond* (London: HMSO; Cmnd 849).

F vs. West Berkshire Health Authority, (1988).

Feinberg, J. (1973) *Social Philosophy* (Englewood Cliffs, New Jersey: Prentice-Hall).

Re B (A Minor) (1987) (Wardship: Sterilisation), 2 All ER.

Rivera, G. (1972) *Willowbrook: A Report On How It Is and Why It Doesn't Have To Be That Way* (New York: Vintage Books).

Tadd, G. V. (1989) *The Sexual Needs of The Mentally Handicapped* (University of Wales: Unpublished Masters Dissertation).

Tadd, W. and Chadwick, R. F. (1989) 'A Bill of Wrongs: Why the Students Bill of Rights Gets it Wrong', *The Professional Nurse*, Sept., pp. 584–6.

Wikler, D. (1979) 'Paternalism and The Mildly Retarded', *Philosophy and Public Affairs*, vol. 8, no. 4, pp. 377–92.

Wolfensburger, W. , cited in A. and M. Craft (1983) *Sex Education and Counselling for Mentally Handicapped People*, p. 25 (Kent: Costello).

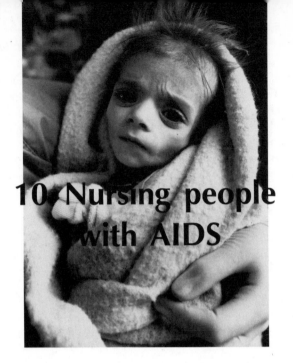

10 Nursing people with AIDS

Introduction

By 1992, it is likely that 30 000 people in the UK will have been diagnosed as suffering from acquired immune deficiency syndrome (AIDS) and, of these, 17 000 will have died (Cox, 1988). In the USA, the picture is even more disconcerting with projections suggesting that 270 000 people will have been diagnosed and 170 000 will require hospitalisation and health care (Watcher, 1986, pp. 177–88).

The impact of such figures on both the health services and the professionals within them will be immense, and yet nurses as primary care givers are still largely unprepared for this alarming addition to their workload. Indeed, it might well be argued that, as yet, society still has to face up to the challenge that AIDS poses not only to health, but also to our lifestyles.

Within the foreseeable future, nursing the patient with AIDS will become part of almost every nurse's practice and it is now that they need to address the ethical issues that will undoubtedly emerge.

AIDS and society

The impact of AIDS on society has largely been one of panic, fuelled no doubt by emotive media reporting such as references to the 'gay plague' and yet, ' . . . the majority of people who are dying of this disease live in the Third World and are not in any sense gay men' (Pierce and VanDeveer, 1988, p. 9).

The fear of contagion that has largely been the public response to AIDS, has resulted in demands for excessive actions such as the tattooing of carriers, the isolation of sufferers and banning those affected from such places as public swimming pools, (Meisenhelder and LaCharite, 1989, pp. 7–9). In 1987 in Bavaria, measures introduced in the name of prevention included the compulsory testing of those suspected of carrying the disease; police powers included forcibly carrying out health checks; foreigners found to be carrying the virus were deported; and there was enforced testing of certain groups such as civil servants, prisoners and prostitutes. If AIDS was discovered then individuals were legally bound to disclose the information to their sexual partners or face heavy fines and prison sentences.

In 1989 the BBC programme, *Taking Liberties*, showed the discrimination taking place today in the UK with regard to the employment of individuals carrying the virus and of people who have friends suffering from the disease.

Such practices raise issues in relation to individual liberty; justice and discrimination; the right to privacy; not to mention the emerging debates about allocation of resources, for both research on AIDS and caring for the sufferers. In this chapter, we will discuss the issues that have a direct bearing on the nurse.

Prejudice

Thiroux (1986, p. 333) defines prejudice as prejudgment often based on biased opinions and frequently leading to discrimination. Whenever we allow prejudice to affect our behaviour towards others, then we can be accused of unfair treatment or acting contrary to the principle of justice.

Prejudicial attitudes towards homosexuality are not new, although the advent of AIDS has certainly rekindled the flames. Charles Stanley, President of the Southern Baptist Convention claimed in the *New York Native*, that AIDS was sent by God to show His displeasure that homosexuality was gaining acceptance in American society (Stanley, 1986, p. 7), and we have heard similar statements reported in the media in this country.

Nurses, like all members of society, are not immune to prejudice, but the danger of judgments such as these in nursing is that they threaten important values such as showing a caring and compassionate response to those in distress. As Loretta Kopelman (1988, pp. 49–55) points out, the punishment concept of disease results in blame being laid at the victim's feet, as the illness is seen as a direct result of being bad or doing bad things. Such attitudes provide a convenient excuse to ignore those in need, 'after all it's *their* fault and so we don't have to help'.

A survey of American nurses involved in caring for AIDS patients showed some disconcerting results which are worth consideration as some reflect the prejudicial nature of nurses' judgments of AIDS patients. Of the 346 respondents from 15 hospitals who took part in the survey 73 per cent were concerned for their own safety, and 46 per cent felt either frightened or angry about caring for AIDS sufferers. When asked whether nurses had the right to refuse to care for AIDS patients, 47 per cent responded positively, although only 7 per cent reported that they had actually refused to give care. An overwhelming majority, 97 per cent, felt that nurses had a right to know a patient's HIV status and some of the comments that respondents made are particularly interesting when considering nurses' attitudes to AIDS:

- 'Being exposed to such a deadly virus is a violation of my rights';
- 'I'm for mandatory testing for all patients';
- 'It's hard to have empathy for someone who's brought the illness on himself' (Brennan, 1988, pp. 60–4).

The sentiment expressed in the final statement is a common response by nurses caring for homosexuals and intravenous drug abusers who have contracted AIDS. Not only does this mirror society's attitude towards drug users, but this group of patients is also particularly difficult to care for, as they frequently feign pain to acquire drugs. Their non-compliance can hamper treatment, and once their condition has improved they may discharge themselves back onto the streets to supply their drug habit (Carpi, 1987, pp. 21–4).

Nursing staff understandably feel that, to some extent, they are wasting their skills, time and valuable resources on a group of people who seem to have little regard for their own welfare. The apparent futility of the situation is believed to be partially responsible for the high burnout rate among nurses caring for such patients (Shelp *et al*, 1986, pp. 144–63).

When we consider that nurses are part of society and therefore share and contribute to society's expression of human fears and failings, such statements are understandable. We need, however, to explore the acceptability of the nurse or any other health professional, translating such attitudes into behaviour towards patients.

For a nurse to adopt prejudicial behaviour is a negation of her professional duty, as nursing, by its very nature, involves a commitment to the service of individual persons, each of whom merits respect as an autonomous individual. No one client or group of clients should be deemed unworthy of nursing care, regardless of the nurse's personal feelings (RCN, 1976).

The nurse chooses to enter the profession and, on registration in the UK, is bound by the Code of Conduct which, in clause 1, demands that she shall 'Act always in such a way as to promote and safeguard the wellbeing and interests of patients or clients' (UKCC, 1984). The Code of Conduct is not written in terms of the best interests of the nurse. Instead, 'The UKCC expects its practitioners to adopt a non-judgmental approach in the exercise of their caring role' (UKCC, 1989).

In America, the American Nurses' Association (ANA), Code for Nurses with Interpretive Statements, expresses similar professional values:

> The need for health care is universal, transcending all national, ethnic, racial, religious, cultural, political, educational, economic, developmental, personality, role and sexual differences. Nursing care is delivered without prejudicial behaviour.
>
> (ANA, 1985)

Anticipating that prejudice and fear would affect the quality of care received by AIDS patients, the ANA's Committee on Ethics issued the following statement regarding prejudice in providing nursing care:

> Nursing is resolute in its perspective that care should be delivered without prejudice, and it makes no allowance for the use of the patient's personal attributes or socio-economic status or the social nature of the health problem as grounds for discrimination.
>
> (ANA, 1986)

Similarly, the medical profession, both in the UK and the USA, has declared its expectation that those requiring medical help should receive unprejudiced attention. The General Medical Council (GMC) in 1988 stated:

> It is unethical for a doctor to withhold treatment from any patient on the basis of a moral judgement that the patients' activities or lifestyle might have contributed to the condition for which treatment was being sought.
>
> (GMC, 1988)

In November 1987, the American Medical Association's (AMA) Council on Ethical and Judicial Affairs (CEJA) published a report entitled 'Ethical Issues Involved in the Growing AIDS Crisis', which asserts that:

> A person who is afflicted with AIDS needs competent, compassionate treatment. Neither those who have the disease nor those who have been infected with the virus should be subjected to discrimination based on fear or prejudice, least of all by members of the health care community.
>
> (AMA, 1987)

Professional obligation

One important consequence of prejudice is the refusal, by nurses and doctors, to treat patients who are either suffering from AIDS or who are sero-positive.

Some nurses have tried to use clause 7 of the Code of Conduct, which is concerned with conscientious objection, to refuse to care for patients who are either suffering from AIDS or who are HIV positive. However, the UKCC in its advisory document, *Exercising Accountability*, has stated that this clause 'does not provide a formula for being selective about the categories of patient or client for whom the practitioner will care (UKCC, 1989).

The UKCC and the RCN have emphasised the nurse's duty to care for the sick and have warned that those who refuse may be called to answer allegations of professional misconduct (UKCC, 1987; RCN, 1987).

A similar stance has been taken by the ANA which, in a publication entitled *Statement Regarding Risk vs. Responsibility in providing Nursing Care*, has stated that 'in most instances, it would be considered morally obligatory for a nurse to give care for an AIDS patient' (ANA, 1986, p. 12).

The medical profession on both sides of the Atlantic has also asserted the doctor's duty to provide care as evidenced by the following quotations:

> it is unethical for a registered medical practitioner to refuse treatment, or investigation for which there are appropriate facilities, on the grounds that the patient suffers or may suffer from a condition which could expose the doctor to personal risk.
>
> (GMC, 1988)

> A physician may not ethically refuse to treat a patient whose condition is within the physician's current realm of competence solely because the patient is sero-positive. The tradition of the American Medical Association, since its organization in 1847, is that: 'when an epidemic prevails, a physician must continue with his labors without regard to the risk of his own health'.
>
> (AMA, 1987)

It appears that members of the nursing and medical professions are expected to assume a certain level of personal risk as part of their professional obligation, although a survey published in the British Medical Journal (BMJ) showed that not only would some general practitioners refuse to care for AIDS patients, but a larger percentage would test the patients without consent, because of concern for their own welfare (Shapiro, 1989, pp. 1563–6).

We need to consider how we are to calculate the levels of personal risk which we could reasonably accept as part of any health professional's duty, as clearly there are limits when risks are very great and cannot be reduced. For example, at the scene of a great tragedy, doctors and nurses are not expected to risk their lives in a fruitless attempt to give care to a hopelessly injured person.

One important consideration will be the patient's need for care and the probability of harm befalling him as a result of a refusal to treat. Another will be the likelihood that treatment will have a beneficial effect upon the patient's condition. The potential for harm to the professional will need to be considered, along with whether any potential for risk can be reduced to an acceptable level. Finally, we need to ascertain whether the risk to the professional is greater than the harm that may befall the patient. It is important to recognise that such a classically described consequentialist argument, however, could also be viewed as an infringement of the practitioner's autonomy, in that the nurse's or doctor's right to choose, is subjugated to the demand to respect the needs of the AIDS sufferer.

If one accepts the arguments above, then where care will meet and satisfy the patient's need and prevent greater harm from occurring there is an obligation for the health professional to provide care. Similarly, even when risks are considered great, if they can be minimised so that the risk of harm to the patient is greater than that to the professional, it is reasonable to expect that the nurse or doctor will fulfil their duty to care.

The cases

Staff attitudes to high risk patients

❝ David had very poor care on the basis of nurses' fear, ignorance and prejudice ❞

During my surgical experience a blind, slightly deaf, middle-aged man named David, was admitted for the drainage of an abscess near the anal sphincter. Because he lived with a younger man and appeared to be very gentle by nature, it was assumed by the qualified nurses that David was a homosexual.

For the whole of his stay in hospital he was kept in a side-ward on his own and there was an obvious reluctance by senior nursing staff and the junior medical staff to spend any time talking to him or discussing his situation. Indeed on more than one occasion I was actively discouraged from going into the side-ward to talk with David, despite the sensory deficits which resulted in him feeling somewhat isolated. Whenever wound dressings or injections were required, a student nurse was always detailed to perform these interventions with strong advice to wear gloves and to take care as 'he probably has AIDS'. I felt that the staff were rude and uncaring in their attitude to this person, who had few visitors and spent many hours alone, sometimes having to wait unnecessarily to have his needs met. Sister even requested the doctor to send bloods for AIDS testing and was quite prepared to do this without informing the patient. I felt ashamed of my colleagues and very sorry for David who I feel had very poor care on the basis of nurses' fear, ignorance and prejudice.

Commentary

As discussed in Chapter 5, justice demands that cases that are similar in relevant respects require equal treatment and, therefore, David's care should have been the same as any other patient with similar needs, regardless of his assumed sexual orientation.

Further, we have seen in our discussion of prejudice that both the nursing and medical professions have asserted that it is not morally permissible for their practitioners to display prejudicial behaviour towards clients or patients. This case demonstrates very adequately the effect of prejudice on the quality of patient care, not to mention the effect on the patient as a person.

Let us now consider the demand that nurses have a right to know a patient's HIV status, in order to safeguard themselves and avoid infection. First, it needs to be emphasised that risks are negligible providing that safe standards of practice are followed. This means that blood and body fluids from all patients must be regarded as posing a potential risk and therefore require that appropriate precautions, such as the wearing of gloves and safe disposal of contaminated needles, are taken.

Second we need to ask, if nurses or any health care professionals are demanding knowledge of the patient's HIV status, does the patient have reciprocal rights? AIDS is no respecter of professional boundaries and already there has been wide media coverage given to the death of a surgeon from the disease. If the concept of rights embraces equality, then it follows from this that patients must have an equal right to demand to know that they are not at risk of being contaminated by a nurse or doctor. Would nurses be prepared to undergo an HIV test to give assurance to an anxious patient?

Accepting such a view could lead us to the edge of a slippery slope where an increasing number of occupational groups would be required to give assurances that their clients would not also be at risk.

It is essential to remember that rights protect important interests. The application of safe standards of care applies to all patients, and negates the need to know which of them are suffering from AIDS. In those cases, it appears that there are not sufficient important interests at stake and, therefore, it is not appropriate for nurses or other health care workers to claim a right to be made aware of the patient's HIV status.

Such demands are even more unrealistic when we consider that the accuracy of screening tests still leaves much to be desired and the value of one test, at any given point, is meaningless. To be able to state categorically that an individual is free of the AIDS virus would require daily testing over a lengthy period of time.

With regard to testing without the patient's consent, it is important to remember the advice given to the nursing profession by the UKCC that:

> nurses, midwives and health visitors expose themselves to the possibility of civil action for damages or criminal charges of assault if they personally take blood specimens, and of aiding and abetting such an assault if they knowingly collude with a doctor in obtaining such specimens.

> (UKCC, 1988)

In addition to any criminal or civil charges, the nurse is also at risk of losing her right to practise.

Undoubtedly, the behaviour of the qualified staff in this scenario is contrary to that expected of professional nurses. This is of particular importance when we consider how influential trained staff are in their capacity as role models to student nurses. It is essential that all nurses, but especially those who have the additional responsibility for educating those new to the profession, display appropriate attitudes and values, especially that which is most fundamental, namely equal respect for all persons.

Refusal to treat

❝ The doctor said he would not be coming up to see Mr Black . . . as he might have AIDS ❞

During my span on a male medical ward on night duty, I had in my care a 40-year-old man who had been admitted the previous afternoon with pyrexia of unknown origin. He had settled for the night, but around 2 a.m. I noticed he was shaking and appeared in great distress.

I knew he had a history of rigors and during his last attack he had suffered a cardiac arrest. Aware of this I telephoned the night sister, as there was only myself and a nursing auxiliary on the ward, the staff nurse having been sent to cover another ward for a while.

Sister told me to inform the doctor which I did immediately as I knew from the report that he had asked to be informed of any further rigors so that bloods could be taken for culture and further investigation.

When the doctor returned my call, I was told that he would not be coming up to see Mr Black as the results of his last blood test indicated that he might have AIDS. He said that further tests would be taken, but at a later date. He finished the conversation by saying, 'Now you won't tell anyone will you?'

I wasn't so stunned at the comments he made, but at the fact that he refused to come and even look at the patient. I had to return to Mr Black. How do you explain such a situation to someone who is shaking uncontrollably and in fear of further arrest? I lied! 'The doctor is very busy at the moment, but he has assured me that everything will be alright and he will be here as soon as he can'.

I remained with Mr Black trying to comfort and calm him while slowly bringing down his temperature and hoping that he would soon fall asleep. During this time the doctor telephoned again and gave the auxiliary the following message for me, 'You won't tell anyone will you?'

When the staff nurse returned I had already resolved to tell her as she was responsible for the patients and I felt she had a right to know. Staff informed the night sister of the events and after contacting the doctor she soon arrived on the ward. She was very angry and I was accused of panicking and spreading confidential information.

Commentary

In the situation described, it is obvious that this patient is in need of care and that appropriate treatment would have the beneficial effect of reducing his temperature and ending the rigors, as well as reducing the likelihood of the potentially fatal consequence of a further arrest. From our discussion of professional obligation it seems that the doctor responsible for Mr Black behaved contrary to professional expectations and as such is morally culpable.

Before leaving this discussion, however, we ought to give some further attention to the behaviour of both the night sister and the doctor. One must question how appropriate it is for a senior nurse to leave a learner to contact a doctor in the middle of the night. Rather, she should visit the ward and ascertain for herself the patient's condition, and then give guidance and support to the student, especially in the absence of a qualified nurse. The sister is apparently oblivious to the position in which this leaves the learner, should the doctor be either difficult or wish to give telephone orders. By choosing these actions, the sister negates her responsibility to both the patient and the student nurse.

The doctor, as we have already discussed, has neglected his duty of care to the patient, who requires treatment either to improve his condition or to prevent harmful consequences. But he then relays information which he deems to be confidential to someone who is not competent to handle it. If the doctor felt that it was important for someone involved in the direct care of the patient to have knowledge of certain facts pertaining to that care, then it seems reasonable to expect that all those involved in such direct care require the information. If only certain personnel need that information, then it is extremely difficult to justify its disclosure to a student and not to a registered practitioner.

It seems unfair that the learner is the only one reprimanded in this situation, first for panicking, although initially the night sister sanctioned alerting the doctor to the patient's deteriorating condition and second, for spreading 'confidential' information. No one offers an explanation as to why it is confidential or why the student alone should have accepted the burden of it or, indeed, why the doctor himself is not guilty of a breach of confidentiality.

This incident shows clearly how much thought the nursing profession needs to give to notions of responsibility and accountability. We cannot relinquish our duties by handing them over as convenient packages to individuals incapable of carrying them out, nor of course can we keep changing the rules when deciding for what we are each responsible.

Conclusion

It is particularly important that nurses address not only the issues involved, but also their attitudes towards this disease and its sufferers. This is particularly important since the government's announcement to proceed with the programme of anonymous, uninformed testing of categories of patients, who have consented to their blood being tested for other reasons.

No doubt the debate that will emerge in the UK as the number of victims rises, will be similar to that currently taking place in the USA, that of public versus private good. Nurses, as the largest group of health care professionals, have a duty to participate in the debate, but their involvement must be on rational, informed and moral grounds, and not a response based on prejudice, fear and self-interest.

References

American Medical Association Council on Ethical and Judicial Affairs (1987) *Ethical Issues Involved In The Growing AIDS Crisis (report A; 1–87)*, pp. 1–4 (Chicago: AMA).

American Nurses' Association (1985) *Code For Nurses With Interpretive Statements*, p. 3 (Kansas City, Mo: ANA).

American Nurses' Association Committee on Ethics (1986) *Statement Regarding Risk vs Responsibility In Providing Nursing Care*, pp. 1–2 (Kansas City, Mo: ANA).

Brennan, L. (1988) 'The Battle Against AIDS: A Report From The Nursing Front', *Nursing*, April, pp. 60–4.

Carpi, J. (1987) 'Treating IV Drug Users – A Difficult Task For Staff', *Aids Patients Care*, Dec, pp. 21–4.

Cox, D. (1988) *Short-term Prediction of HIV Infection In England And Wales. Report of a Working Group* (London: HMSO).

General Medical Council (1988) *HIV Infection and AIDS: The Ethical Considerations* (London: GMC).

Kopelman, L. (1988) 'The Punishment Concept of Disease', in C. Pierce and D. VanDeveer (eds), *AIDS: Ethics and Public Policy*, pp. 49–55 (Belmont, California: Wadsworth).

Meisenhelder, J. B. and LaCharite, C. (1989) 'Fear of Contagion: The Public Response to AIDS', *Image*, vol. 21, No.1, pp. 7–9.

Pierce, C. and VanDeever, D. (eds) (1988) *AIDS: Ethics and Public Policy*, pp. 1–27 (Belmont, California: Wadsworth).

Royal College of Nursing (1976) *Code of Professional Conduct – A Discussion Document* (London: RCN).

Royal College of Nursing (1987) *AIDS: Nursing Guidelines* (London: RCN).

Shapiro, J. A. (1989) 'General Practitioners Attitudes Towards AIDS and Their Perceived Information Needs', *British Medical Journal*, vol. 298, pp. 1563–6.

Shelp, E. E. *et al*, (1986) *AIDS – Personal Stories in Pastoral Perspectives*, pp. 144–63 (New York: Pilgrim Press).

Stanley, C. (1986) as quoted in *New York Native*, Feb. 10–16, p. 7.

Thiroux, J. P. (1986) *Ethics Theory and Practice* (New York: Macmillan).

United Kingdom Central Council for Nurses, Midwives and Health Visitors (1984) *Code of Professional Conduct for the Nurse, Midwife and Health Visitor, 2nd ed.* (London: UKCC).

United Kingdom Central Council for Nurses, Midwives and Health Visitors (1987) *Aids, Testing, Treatment and Care. PC/87/02* (London: UKCC).

United Kingdom Central Council for Nurses, Midwives and Health Visitors (1988) *AIDS and HIV Infection. PC/88/03* (London: UKCC).

United Kingdom Central Council for Nurses, Midwives and Health Visitors (1989) *Exercising Accountability* (London: UKCC).

Watcher, R. (1986) 'Sounding Board: The Impact of Acquired Immunodeficiency Syndrome on Medical Residency Training', *New England Journal of Medicine*, vol. 314, pp. 177–80.

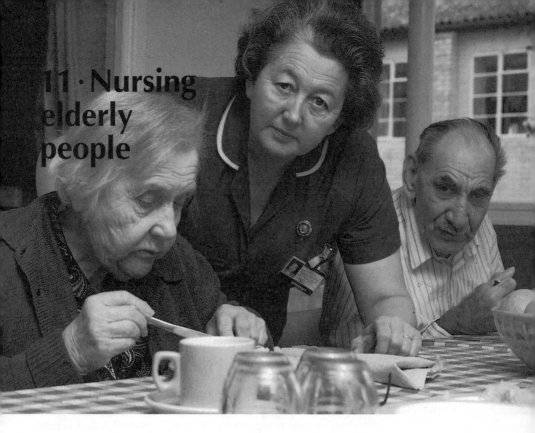

11 · Nursing elderly people

Introduction

The proportion of elderly people in the population is growing fast, and they are major consumers of health care. In addition, they require and will require for the foreseeable future a large number of carers and, as Muyskens points out, in this area of health care it is nurses who will be required, rather than physicians. 'For the ailing aged and the chronically ill, the skills of the physician are really ancillary to the caring functions of the nurse' (Muyskens, 1982, p. 100).

Despite these facts, there is a general reluctance to work in this area (Feldbaum and Feldbaum, 1981). It has an unglamorous image, there is little in the way of spectacular success and the work may seem hard and unrewarding. In the context of a shortage of nurses generally, the American College of Health Care Administrators has suggested positive steps to enhance the image of this area of work, pointing out that it is 'an opportunity to practise 'total patient/resident care' and make a difference to the quality of the elderly person's life' (Tourigny and Fiore, 1988). Much of the care of the elderly, being long-term, has as its object 'residents' rather than 'patients', but for the sake of simplicity we shall use the term 'patients' throughout.

Some writers have pointed beyond facts about the nature of the care setting, to features of our society that make it uncomfortable for us to confront the sufferings of elderly people. In a society that values the pursuit of individual self-interest, and where success is measured in material terms, the decline of old age must appear as a failure. Young people may find it difficult, if not impossible, to come to terms with, or to imagine their own inevitable ageing and death. So, working with old people may be feared as a reminder of certain unpleasant truths. One of the things a nurse may need to confront is how she feels about the old, and why? This introduces us to our first issue, that of ageism.

Ageism

The term ageism was coined by Robert Butler in 1968 to describe the systematic stereotyping of and discrimination against older people (quoted in Cole, 1983, p. 34).

In Chapter 5 we saw that to discriminate against a person on the grounds of an irrelevant characteristic is unjust. It is argued by anti-ageists that to discriminate against someone simply on the grounds of age is an example of such injustice, because age is, in itself, an irrelevant characteristic.

If age is irrelevant, how come ageism is so widespread? Ageist beliefs do not, of course, openly suggest that people should be discriminated against simply because they are old: on the contrary, age is associated in the mind of the ageist with certain other characteristics which may be thought to justify a dismissive attitude. This is the phenomenon of the stereotyping of old age. For example, one such stereotype portrays people of very advanced years as confused:

> The elderly person is considered to have regressed to a state in which he or she is no longer in touch with reality, no longer possessed of a clear grasp of his or her own interests, and thus stands in need of some form of guardianship.
>
> (Kleinig, 1983, p. 167)

The anti-ageist strategy is to show that these stereotypes are just that – stereotypes – and tell us nothing about any particular individual. What we have to remember, according to the anti-ageist, are the features that elderly people share with everyone else – physical, emotional, intellectual and spiritual (Gunter et al, 1979).

One suggestion is that even to use terms such as 'the elderly' is dangerous. It implies that elderly people can be treated as a group, without regard for their individual differences. It may, however, be harmless enough to use the term, if we avoid the possible unwelcome implications, but what do we mean by it?

The elderly

When does an individual become an elderly person? To some extent this is an impossible question to answer, similar to the questions about when personhood begins, or when middle age starts. It is also clearly relative to social context. In general, contemporary Western society fixes on the age of 65 years as the onset of elderly status (Bandman and Bandman, 1985, p. 210). In recent times, however, this has proved insufficient. With increased longevity has come a tendency to divide the elderly into the young elderly and the advanced elderly (Bandman and Bandman, 1985). One potential danger here is that it is this latter group who will be designated frail and senile, whether or not this is true of particular individuals, while to the young group will be assigned the image of self-sufficiency, material comfort, and 'grey power'.

This more recent image of a certain group of elderly people can be just as dangerous as the old one. To think of a group as being without need of help, as self-sufficient, may be just as misguided as to write off a group as senile and confused, in need of caring others to take charge of their lives. Both stereotypes may mask the problems of individuals.

It is the task of the anti-ageist, then, to expose these stereotypes and to urge that elderly people should be treated as individuals. Some writers have been concerned that anti-ageism may go too far in holding that elderly people are just the same as everyone else, with the result that real needs and relevant differences may be overlooked. Thus, Dan Callahan argues that there are many generalisations about the elderly that are both inoffensive and true. For example, that people over the age of 65 years have greater health care needs than those under 65 years of age (Callahan, 1987, pp. 122–3). To accept this need not blind us to the variations between individuals.

Respect for the individual

How do our moral principles apply with regard to the elderly? It is common (though perhaps less nowadays than it used to be) to hear people talk about 'showing respect for one's elders'. In this sense of showing respect, the suggestion is that the elderly *as a group* deserve to be shown deference, on the grounds of their greater experience and wisdom. Some see it as a loss in our society that this tradition has been undermined. This is not, however, what is meant by the application of the principle of respect for the elderly. It involves concern for the common humanity of the individual patient.

In the case of the elderly, particularly for those in long-term residential care, respect for the individual person takes on particular significance, for in such an institutional setting it is remarkably easy for patients to lose their individuality. Patients are vulnerable to being swallowed up by their surroundings and by the systems of the care setting. Practical steps that nurses can take to counteract this trend include encouraging relatives to bring in the elderly person's personal possessions. Muyskens emphasises the importance of security and belonging to which this may contribute (Muyskens, 1982, pp. 105–6), and to security and belonging we might add dignity.

The case studies will show us how easy it may be to threaten the dignity of elderly people in the course of everyday care.

Autonomy and the elderly person

When the principle of autonomy is considered, elderly people, though adults, may suffer from at least two disadvantages. First, because of stereotyping there may be a tendency to classify an elderly person as incompetent, or to reject the presumption that operates in the case of competent adults that the exercise of autonomy is usually in their best interests. Second, there have been some suggestions in the recent literature that elderly persons' expressions of their wishes, though competent, may be 'inauthentic'.

Authenticity

Should we respect the choice of a competent adult, even if that choice appears to be out of character, that is, inauthentic? Some would say no, holding that:

> In full measure, autonomy is the active expression of human
> identity, intention and history . . .. Authentic
> autonomy . . . consists in choices and behaviour that are deeply
> in character, that flow from past moral career and ethical style,
> as well as from present values and immediate self-shaping.
>
> (Collopy, 1988, p. 14)

In the context of care for elderly patients, the implication is that we should ask ourselves whether a given choice is in accord with what we know of that person's past character and values.

At first sight this seems open to gross abuse. How is it possible for a carer, or even a relative, to assert that he knows a person's character so intimately that he can be confident in making a judgement that a certain decision is authentic or inauthentic? For it is a fact of life that people's values change as a result of experience. A person who, while healthy, has argued rationally in favour of euthanasia for the terminally ill may change his mind when in that situation.

On the other hand, we are familiar with the sort of situation in which we say of someone that he does not mean what he says because 'He's not himself'. So maybe there is something in the notion of authenticity. Collopy argues, further, that the notion of authenticity may operate not only as a threat but also as a protective mechanism. For a decision that proves unpopular with the caring staff may, nevertheless, be supported on the grounds that it was exactly the sort of decision we might expect Mr X to make, knowing his past character.

On balance, however, given the temptations to paternalism in the case of elderly people, the danger of abuse seems to outweigh the potential for benefit. It denies the possibility of change and, as Wetle has pointed out, autonomy of the elderly may be subtly disregarded by caring staff, and this needs to be avoided. He notes how the physician, for example, may automatically consult adult children rather than the elderly person himself (Wetle, 1985, p. 259). Moreover, if authenticity is introduced only in the elderly care setting, but not for, say, 40-year-old adults, then we have additional reasons for being suspicious.

Negative and positive autonomy

Collopy makes another distinction which may be useful when speaking of autonomy and the elderly, and that is between negative and positive autonomy. To respect Mr X's autonomy by simply refraining from interfering in his choices is to respect it in a negative way, i.e. by not doing anything. It is possible, however, to take positive action to restore a patient's autonomy. Under this heading fall the activities involved in encouraging self-reliance, mobility and independence.

This is a very important aspect of care for elderly people. It is well known that long-term residential care can easily foster dependency. According to one stereotype, dependency is assumed to be a natural feature of old age (Wetle, 1985, p. 263). To counteract this, it is argued by Muyskens, among others, that 'the morally proper role for the nurse is to help the client, wherever possible, to help himself or herself' (Muyskens, 1982, p. 105). The disadvantages of this are practical: it is time-consuming for staff who are already pushed to the limit. Hence, there may be temptations, for example, to use restraints too readily. As Collopy points out, to support a positive interpretation of what is involved in respecting an elderly person's autonomy raises the problem of the extent of our expectations of carers. 'Given scarce resources and multiple, competing claims on them, caregivers cannot face absolutely open-ended obligations' (Collopy, 1988, p. 17). It may be difficult to know how best to allocate the time one has.

Justice and the elderly

In allocating her time, the nurse faces questions not only of efficiency but also of justice. This arises with every group of patients, as we have seen, and in the case of the elderly, as with the others, it is unjust to allocate one's time on irrelevant criteria, for example, to ignore a patient's needs because he is 'difficult' or a nuisance.

These are the questions of allocation that are most likely to concern the nurse at the bedside. But the nursing profession as a whole, along with every other section of society, is going to be increasingly faced with the larger scale problems of allocation of health care resources to the elderly in the future. Insofar as they make up an identifiable segment of the population, the elderly constitute only one group among others, and their claims for resources inevitably compete with others, such as children and parents of young children. Questions are now being asked about what we owe the elderly, what resources should be made available to them, and suggestions are being made that it will be necessary to 'set limits' to their care (Callahan, 1987).

The consequences of this trend might be that old people will come to be seen more and more as a burden on society, and receive increasingly poor treatment. Callahan argues, however, that this need not be the case if we change our attitudes to old age. He suggests that it may genuinely not be in the best interests of the elderly to be subjected to a great deal of invasive medicine, but it is not sufficient simply to stop providing it. Rather than encourage medicine to strive heroically to keep people alive beyond a 'natural lifespan', society should be looking for ways of giving meaning to old age, and valuing a medicine which concentrates on the relief of suffering for those at the end of their lives, thereby improving the quality of their lives.

The nursing profession has the opportunity and the responsibility to join in the search for answers to these questions. Should elderly people have the right to exactly the same treatment as everyone else, or should we consider it relevant that some people have already lived a natural lifespan? Should medical research concentrate less on life-prolonging technology and more on chronic problems, such as incontinence and pressure sores?

What is important is that such decisions should be made on criteria that are relevant and just; that we do not decide to give elderly people inferior treatment because we think that old people are in some sense less valuable than others. If decisions about allocations of resources are made, at a social level, which result in a change in the sort of health care made available to elderly people, the nurse at the bedside still has the obligation to act in the best interests of the patient within the constraints of the resources available, showing respect, maintaining dignity, and allowing room for autonomy.

The cases

Nasogastric feeding

❛ *The staff did not agree with wasting time helping slow people* ❜

In my first year as a student nurse, on a very busy acute geriatric ward, the staff did not agree with wasting time helping slow people who could not feed themselves. They found it quicker just to pass a nasogastric tube and give them a feed by this method, even when they could swallow and feed with assistance and time.

Commentary

When there is serious understaffing, it is understandable that nursing staff feel they have all too little time to allocate to patients. It might even be argued that, if all the patients on the ward are treated in the same way, then this is fair and just: no one person is singled out for inferior treatment. On the contrary, every person on the ward is fed by a nasogastric tube.

There are several objections, however, to this line of argument. First, according to the account given by the student nurse, this ward policy is not formulated in the interests of the patients, but in the interests of the nursing staff. That may be understandable, but it is not in accord with the Code of Conduct (UKCC, 1984).

Second, there is not, in fact, a just allocation of resources here. Some of the patients will need feeding nasogastrically, but we are told explicitly that others do not. So, no account is taken of individual needs or of the relevant differences between patients. As we have seen, to treat people in the same way, as a group, when there are in fact relevant differences between them is unjust.

Third, no attempt is made to respect autonomy in this case study. When patients are capable of doing something for themselves, to deny them that opportunity is to reinforce dependence and further erode what capacity for autonomy they have (Chadwick and Russell, 1989). We saw above that it is difficult to be precise about the extent to which autonomy should positively be developed, but the actions described in this case may be doing actual harm.

To force someone to have a nasogastric tube inserted when it is unnecessary is an assault on human dignity, showing no respect for the individual. Would any one of the nurses be content that it should be done to them, if they were capable of managing alone? This is a good test to apply (Hare, 1981) and shows us that it is not even necessary to appeal to abstract notions of human dignity in assessing the morality of this case: we simply have to think about how we would feel in this situation, and of the feelings of the elderly persons subjected to it. On the grounds of both the autonomy principle and the consequences for the patient, then, the action is not in the best interests of the patient.

The incontinent patient

❬ When cleaning her up nurse A was very rude and unkind to her ❭

I was working with nurse A in an elderly care ward one morning, looking after a 70-year-old woman who was very obese. We went to put the woman on the commode at about 11.00 a.m., but found it rather difficult, and the woman was unable to help us very much. Nurse A was shouting at her and pulling on her arms, telling her not to be so lazy, which was making the woman very distressed. Nurse A then said to leave her and sat her back in the chair.

Within an hour the poor woman had been incontinent and I went back to tell nurse A. When cleaning her up nurse A was very rude and unkind to her, being rough to the point of hitting her on the arm. I was told not to put any underwear on her and she was sat back in the chair with only a blanket to cover her lower parts.

Commentary

Incontinence is common in an elderly care setting. It does not raise any of the so-called life and death issues of health care ethics, but the way it is dealt with can make an enormous difference to the lives of those affected. This is an example of the way in which nursing ethics is concerned with everyday matters and with making people's lives more acceptable to them.

To have to deal with incontinence continually may, of course, become a source of irritation for the nursing staff. However, it is clearly unacceptable, according to the Code of Conduct, to take this out on the patients. It is difficult to see how the actions described above could conceivably count as being in the best interests of the patient.

In terms of ethics, we could once more invoke the principle of respect for persons. This urges us to look beyond the 'nuisance' of the incontinence itself to the humanity of the persons who suffer from it, an humanity that they share with the carer. To them their incontinence may be humiliating; to treat them like naughty children only increases their humiliation, and violates the principle of respect for persons.

We saw above the importance of enabling elderly persons to retain their own identity, and noted the part that personal belongings can play in this. To deprive a person of their clothes is a symbol of an almost total lack of respect, and a way of depriving them of their individuality and of damaging their self-image.

Apart from these considerations, if we look at the consequences of the kind of attitude described above, we can see how counter-productive it can be. For to make elderly patients feel guilty about their incontinence is unlikely to improve their condition.

The right to refuse intervention

❝ *The consultant insisted the staff nurse tie his arms to the cotsides* ❞

One incident during my training occurred when a 90-year-old man was admitted to the ward with dehydration and weight loss. He had recently lost his wife and had no other relatives or friends still living, and had decided to give up living by starving himself. He repeatedly removed IVI's and nasogastric (NG) feeds, refusing fluids and diet. To prevent him pulling the NG tube out the consultant insisted the staff nurse tie his arms to the cotsides. I thought that we should not force people to accept treatment if they did not want it. Although this man was 90 years of age, he was fully mentally alert. Other nurses on the ward agreed with me but no one said anything to medical staff for a long time. One day his arms were untied so that he could be turned and were 'accidentally' left untied afterwards.

Commentary

The first issue here is that of the autonomy of the patient. If it is his considered wish to refuse all forms of nourishment, so that he will die, should that wish be respected? We are told that he is fully alert mentally, so there is no evidence that he is incompetent to make a decision. What of the question of authenticity? Even if we believed that this notion was helpful, in this case it would be difficult to appeal to it, as there appears to be no one available who has known the patient well enough to tell us whether this decision is 'in character'.

The principle of autonomy, then, would urge us in the direction of respecting the patient's wish to die, but the consultant is against that. On what grounds?

It goes against the whole tradition of medical ethics to stand by and let somebody starve to death. On one view there is a sharp difference between 'medical' treatment and feeding, and while it may be permissible to cease the former, to stop feeding would be inhumane. As Callahan points out, to deny food 'will be the specific cause of death, and therefore will have the appearance of direct killing rather than mere allowing to die' (Callahan, 1987, p. 187). On another view, however, artificial feeding, at least, is a medical intervention and, if there are ever grounds for ceasing to treat, there may be grounds for ceasing to feed.

But whatever the consultant's grounds for his action, what are the particular problems for the nursing staff? It is a nurse who receives the order to restrain the patient. If she disagrees with it, the problems discussed in Chapter 4, of obedience to the doctor's authority, arise. But let us suppose that that particular issue is resolved in the nurse's mind, so that she thinks that it is necessary to defy an order if she sincerely believes it to be wrong. So, it is a nurse who 'accidentally' leaves the patient's arm untied so that he can pull out his feeding tubes. The nurse says 'I thought that we should not force people to accept treatment if they did not want it'. Is she right?[1]

One argument against respecting the autonomy of the patient in this case might be that autonomy conflicts with what is in the best interests of the patient, and the nurse must always act in the patient's best interests. Surely it cannot be in his best interests to go without food with the result that he will die and have no future interests at all?

The American Nurses' Association Guidelines on Withdrawing or Withholding Food and Fluid say:

> The benefits of life and health from receiving food and fluid are so clear that, especially for those in the health professions (and perhaps most especially for nurses), there is a generally unambiguous moral duty to provide them.
>
> (ANA, 1988, pp. U1123–4)

So can it ever be right to refrain from feeding him? The ANA's answer to this is yes, holding that it is both morally and legally permissible for nurses to respect the refusal of food and fluid by competent patients. Patients have certain rights which entitle them to refuse food and fluids. These rights protect very deep-seated interests, such as the interest in being respected as an individual person with a life of one's own.

The ANA, however, cautions that it may not be in the patient's best interests where an apparent respect for autonomy conceals indifference to the patient's welfare. It may be a temporary depression which produces a wish to die, and it could therefore be dangerous to be too quick to act on that wish. 'It is the patient's *reasons* which . . . are pivotal in determining what the nurse should do' (ANA, 1988, p. U1124).

This point is very important. To pay lip-service to the principle of autonomy sometimes masks a lack of concern (Chadwick and Russell, 1989). What the American guidelines suggest is that a patient's decision to give up taking food may be reversible, and that the nurse has an obligation to attempt to reverse it before accepting that the decision to die is final.

In coming to the conclusion that it is final, how relevant is the patient's age? It is not relevant in the sense that it justifies the view that his life is valueless and therefore not worth saving. It may be relevant in our acceptance of his reasons for his decision. He may feel that he has what Callahan calls a 'full biography' (Callahan, 1987, p. 172). If a man of 40 years of age had lost his nearest and dearest in a terrible accident, we might expect him to start again and build a new life for himself, though realising it would be difficult. But there comes a point beyond which this becomes rather unrealistic. It is true that at 90 years of age there are prospects of many enjoyable experiences, but to compel a person to go on living by force-feeding, because we think that his life is still worthwhile, when it has lost all meaning for him, could be cruel. Perhaps we need in health care something like Dan Callahan's concept of a natural life span, beyond which there is no obligation to prolong life, but only to relieve suffering[2] (Callahan, 1987, p. 137). On this view it does not necessarily involve a discriminatory attitude towards the elderly to think that a death at the age of 90 years is less of a tragedy than a death at 40 years of age.

If these arguments are accepted, there is no conflict between the principles of autonomy and best interests, and the old man's wish should be respected. There would still be a question about whether it should be done in such a surreptitious way, by 'accidentally' leaving off the restraints. It is worth asking for whose benefit this is done; who is to be convinced by this form of action. Is it the consultant, who gave the order to keep the restraints on? Is it a form of self-deception, in order to help the nursing staff feel that they were not responsible for the patient's death? Does it display a fear of social attitudes, a worry that there would be a public outcry if this came to light? Or is it a genuine attempt to give the power of decision back to the old man at the end?

There is yet another dimension to this case. Although, as far as this patient is concerned, it might appear to be justifiable to allow the patient to die, there are of course questions about the consequences for other patients, and for society as a whole, if it is thought acceptable for people to go into hospital and be allowed to starve to death. The extent to which the nurse at the bedside has the time to reflect on such matters is limited, but what is needed is greater public discussion about the circumstances, if any, in which we think it is permissible to withhold food and fluids. It is for the nursing profession as a whole to contribute to such discussions. Without such debate the nurse at the bedside faces dilemmas unprepared and without support.

Conclusion

We have seen how the principles of respect for persons, autonomy and justice have special application in the context of care of the elderly. The most important questions for nurses relate to the value we place on the elderly, especially in the context of demands to reduce their share of the health care cake. As persons they have lives that are of equal value to those of other persons, but this basic equality should not make us overlook real differences between their needs and those of other groups.

> this kind of medical care requires skills and understanding which go well beyond technical knowledge . . . [T]hat . . . health care workers must be prepared to spend time in talking with the elderly, and giving of themselves to them, is a prime duty.
>
> (Callahan, 1987, pp. 78–9)

Notes

[1] In assessing this case it would be useful to know how the old man came to be admitted to hospital, and whether that, too, was against his will. In the UK, under the National Assistance Act of 1948 there is a power to take old people into hospital whether or not they are incompetent, but this power is rarely used. If he was voluntarily admitted, then it might be argued that there was an implied consent from him to accept care.

[2] Although, we suspect he might take a different view in this case, as he is against assisted suicide for the elderly.

References

American Nurses Association (1988) 'Guidelines on Withdrawing or Withholding Food and Fluid', *Biolaw*, vol. 2, pp. U1123–26.

Bandman, E. L. and Bandman, B. (1985) *Nursing Ethics in the Life Span* (Norwalk: Appleton-Century Crofts).

Callahan, D. (1987) *Setting Limits: Medical Goals in an Aging Society* (New York: Simon & Schuster).

Chadwick, R. and Russell, J. (1989) 'Hospital discharge of frail elderly people: social and ethical considerations in the discharge decision-making process, *Ageing and Society*, vol. 9, pp. 277–95.

Cole, T. (1983) 'The "enlightened" view of aging', *Hastings Center Report*, vol. 13, pp. 34–40.

Collopy, B. (1988) 'Autonomy in long-term care: some crucial distinctions, *The Gerontologist*, vol. 28, Suppl. issue, pp. 10–17.

Feldbaum, E. G. and Feldbaum, M. B. (1981) 'Caring for the elderly: who dislikes it least', *Journal of Health Politics, Policy and Law*, vol. 6, pp. 62–72.

Gunter, L. M., Heckman, L. M., Moser, D. H. and Fasano, M. A. (1979) 'Issues and Ethics in Geriatric Nursing', *Journal of Gerontological Nursing*, vol. 5, pp. 15–20.

Hare, R. M. (1981) *Moral Thinking: Its Levels, Methods and Point* (Oxford: Oxford University Press).

Kleinig, J. (1983) *Paternalism* (Manchester: Manchester University Press).

Muyskens, J. L. (1982) *Moral Problems in Nursing: a Philosophical Investigation* (Totowa: Rowman & Littlefield).

Tourigny, A. W. and Fiore, L. (1988) 'Nurses: our endangered species', *Journal of Long-Term Care Administration*, vol. 16, pp. 19–21.

United Kingdom Central Council for Nursing, Midwifery and Health Visiting (1984) *Code of Professional Conduct for the Nurse, Midwife and Health Visitor*, 2nd ed. (London: UKCC).

Wetle, T. T. (1985) 'Ethical aspects of decision-making for and with the elderly' in M. B. Kapp, H. E. Pies and A. E. Doudera (eds) *Legal and Ethical Aspects of Health Care for the Elderly*, pp. 258–67 (Ann Arbor: Health Admin. Press).

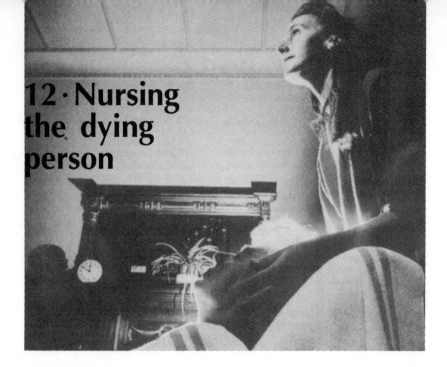

12 · Nursing the dying person

Introduction

The issues surrounding death and dying are many, ranging from those that arise in relation to organ transplantation, such as how death is to be defined and when is it thought to occur, to those concerning how the dying person is to be treated. The focus of this chapter will be on the problems raised in the latter category, as these represent the concerns of many nurses in their day-to-day work.

Perceptions of death

The inevitability of death has never been more challenged than it is today. The 20th century has seen rapid advances in medical technology with the result that frequently death is no longer viewed as a natural process, but as an enemy that must be forced into retreat whenever possible. This is evidenced in much of the literature on death and dying; 'The oft heard complaint that no-one dies anymore – they arrest, must be taken seriously' (Melia, 1987, pp. 43–5), and 'A patient can commit no more grievous offense in a university hospital than to die' (Caroline, 1972, pp. 655–7). Also, over recent years, we have seen the advent of cryogenics, particularly in North America, where individuals are willing to pay vast sums of money to have their bodies frozen into what they hope will be a state of suspended animation from which, at some point in the future, they will hopefully re-emerge and resume their lives.

This seems to point to the fact that for many people, death is viewed as an evil. 'Death is never a good . . .. The whole history of western medicine has always seen it as an evil to be fought and struggled with . . . ' (Riga, 1989, pp. 53–62). With the prevalence of such views, it is easy to understand why doctors and nurses feel the need to struggle, often against all odds to preserve life, and to feel that they have failed when the inevitable happens.

It is important to recognise this, as the way that we care for the critically ill or dying person may well be shaped by how we view death. In considering what it is that is bad about death, Thomas Nagel argues that it is not the state of being dead or not existing, that is objectionable, but that it is the loss of life itself (Nagel, 1986, pp. 9–18). This means that to determine why such great importance is placed on postponing death, it is necessary to consider what is valuable about being alive.

The value of life

For some such as Schweitzer, all life was sacred. For religious believers the sanctity of life stems from the view that it is God-given and human life is particularly valuable, as man was created in God's image and possesses an immortal soul.

This does not, of course, mean that those who do not hold religious beliefs claim that life has no intrinsic value. Indeed most of us feel strongly that killing is wrong and society exacts the severest of punishments for convicted murderers. It does not follow, however, that the sanctity of life doctrine is an absolute one.

There are extreme circumstances when it might be deemed necessary to take a life, for example in self-defence or in war time, and the extremeness of such examples merely serves to illustrate the value that we place on life.

We need to exercise some caution here as many philosophers have argued that life itself has no intrinsic value, but that there are certain characteristics and qualities which render life valuable (Bayles, 1980, pp. 2226–30; Glover, 1977, pp. 45–7). These discussions have serious implications in a health care context, when decisions are taken daily about who will live and die, and about how people are to die, especially when the basis for such decision-making is consideration of the quality of life.

Quality of life

Nurses and doctors frequently use the quality of an individual's life as a justification for deciding whether a particular course of treatment is optional or obligatory, or when resources are scarce, who should have them. The obvious difficulties of this approach are first, how to judge the quality of a particular life and second, to decide who will be the judge.

No one definition of the quality of life is universally acceptable, despite the many attempts of various philosophers. Historically it has been associated with happiness, pleasure or the absence of pain, but as Aristotle points out this too is of little help

> when it comes to saying in what happiness consists, opinions differ . . . and often the same person changes his opinion. When he falls ill he says that it is health, and when he is hard up he say that it is money.
>
> Aristotle, 1980, 1095a, pp. 20–5)

The notion of the quality of life is a 'loose concept', as it means different things to different people and different things to the same person at different times in their life. The danger of its application in health care contexts arises from the two ways in which it may be used. A common sentiment expressed by nurses, is that we should promote quality of life rather than quantity. One way of interpreting this is that health care professionals should concern themselves primarily with what can truly benefit the patient, a sentiment which we would agree is morally commendable. A second interpretation is that some lives lack quality and therefore we need not strive to sustain them or we may even take steps to end them.

We have already seen this interpretation applied to the handicapped neonate, when food is withheld on the basis that the infant's quality of life will be poor.

McCormick (1974, pp. 172–6) suggested that the potential for human relationships would serve as a useful criterion to guide quality of life decisions. One might wish to ask, however, where does this leave the comatose person or someone inflicted with Alzheimer's disease? Edith Schaeffer, while not disregarding totally the use of such considerations in medical decision-making, warns us of the dangers ' . . . Once it becomes acceptable to decide that the quality of life is no longer worthwhile, just abort it.' (Schaeffer, 1978, pp. 216–7).

As deliberations about the quality of life relate to individual persons, then the best judge must be the person whose life is being considered. Therefore, whenever possible nurses and doctors should fully involve patients and clients in discussions about whether or not a particular course of action would promote a better quality of life.

The difficulties arise when the patient cannot, for whatever reason, decide on his own behalf and a quotation cited by David Lamb (1985, p. 109) identifies the dangers inherent in this position:

If the physician presumes to take into consideration in his work whether a life has value or not, the consequences are boundless and the physician becomes the most dangerous man in the state.

(Dr C. Hufeland, 1762–1836)

Having identified some of the difficulties in trying to decide the quality of life, let us now consider our responses to the question of euthanasia. Although it is not yet legalised, it is certainly openly tolerated in some European countries, namely Holland, and in this country it is a subject of great public and professional interest.

Euthanasia

Translated from the Greek, euthanasia literally means an easy or happy death, and it was not until quite recently that its usage changed to encompass ' . . . the act or practice of bringing about an easy and painless death' (Beauchamp, 1975, p. 57).

In order to assist thinking about this complex issue various categories of euthanasia are described. Harris describes three categories hinged on the notion of consent:

- *Voluntary euthanasia*, when an individual consciously requests that his or her life is ended;
- *Involuntary euthanasia* which occurs against the wishes of the individual;
- *Non-voluntary euthanasia* where consent of the individual is lacking, for example the person may be unconscious, incompetent or below the age of consent (Harris, 1985, p. 82–3).

Before discussing the implications of these categories, we need to take account of a further distinction which can be made in relation to the various types of euthanasia. This distinction focuses on the involvement of the agent. *Active euthanasia* is that which is brought about by a direct action, that is 'killing'. On the other hand, *passive euthanasia* is a case of 'allowing to die'. Although active euthanasia is frowned upon by most practitioners in this country, there is generally an acceptance in health care settings that passive euthanasia can more readily be justified.

We need, however, to be aware that there is great philosophical debate about whether there are morally relevant differences between killing and letting die. Some considerations frequently cited include, intentions and motives, withholding and withdrawing treatment, acts and omissions and positive and negative responsibilities. Although it is not possible to fully explore this debate within this chapter, a brief discussion of some of the above may be of value.

Letting die

We need first to challenge the commonly held assumption that 'letting die' is an invariably benign and peaceful process, chosen because it alone best serves the demands of beneficence and non-maleficence. No doubt this is partly due to the emotiveness of the term itself – 'letting die' with its implication that the patient is in some way already trying to die and all that is required is not to impede him on his journey. For example, Melia states:

> It is perhaps unhelpful to consider cases of passive euthanasia, where the patient is 'allowed to die' without undue medical intervention, under the euthanasia banner, albeit qualified by the label 'passive', for it raises more concerns than are perhaps necessary. Such treatment comes within the principles of beneficence and non-maleficence, and to introduce the notion of euthanasia and its 'putting to death' connotations complicates the business in an unhelpful way.
>
> (Melia, 1989, p. 53)

This depends of course on what we agree will count as passive. Already we have seen the term 'allowing to die' applied to the withholding of food from handicapped infants, but it has also been applied to the withdrawing of treatment, as in 1985 when a middle-aged man in an Oxford hospital was removed from a renal dialysis programme on the grounds that his quality of life was such that he could not benefit (*Guardian*, Jan 8, 1985).

According to Lamb (1988, p. 67) the first case constitutes one of passive non-voluntary euthanasia, while the second amounts to one of passive involuntary euthanasia. Not all philosophers would agree however with this classification. John Ladd (1979) and Paul Ramsey (1970) both allude to the notion that withdrawing treatment already commenced constitutes active euthanasia, whereas withholding treatment is routinely interpreted as allowing to die.

This distinction is particularly relevant in intensive care units where, in admitting difficult cases, such as the patient with long-standing chronic obstructive airways disease or those with severe head injuries, great debate precedes the initiation of artificial ventilation, as this may create the further problem of deciding to withdraw or discontinue artificial ventilation at a later date.

We need to be aware that judgements about either commencement or pursuance of a course of treatment depend, to a large extent, upon the type of treatment under consideration and the nature of the disease or illness suffered. Also, as Beauchamp and Childress (1983, p. 115) emphasise, it is frequently necessary to initiate treatment to establish either a diagnosis or to estimate a prognosis and it would therefore be unjust to penalise health professionals and accuse them of killing patients, when they had been intending to act in an individual's best interests.

Michael Bayles (1983) emphasises the need for a clearer definition of the term 'treatment' when attempting to determine the acceptability of either withholding or withdrawing it, for, as the following shows, a wide variety of treatment classifications exist. These range from those that are palliative and function to increase comfort, to those that are curative, such as the surgical correction of structural defects or the administration of an antibiotic for a bacterial infection. Another class of treatments maintain health by ameliorating the effects of deficiencies in either bodily secretions or homeostatic mechanisms, as for example the administration of hormonal therapies or anti-hypertensive agents. Some treatments impede the progress of a disease, such as anti-inflammatory agents as used in rheumatism, or chemotherapy for certain types of cancer. Finally, some treatments, such as the use of artificial ventilation, may be classed as supportive as they are used when major bodily functions have failed and require artificial maintenance.

Let us imagine that an individual has contracted pneumonia and the doctor either withholds antibiotics or having commenced them, withdraws the therapy after 24 hours and the patient dies. In either case, it is reasonable to say that he has let his patient die of pneumonia; the statements do not sound odd nor are they contradictions.

Whenever treatment for a life-threatening condition cures, maintains health, retards disease or sustains life, it can be said that the withdrawing or withholding of such treatment will result in the patient's death. The simple distinction between withholding and withdrawing treatment is unhelpful, therefore, in determining whether or not there are morally relevant differences between killing and letting die or active and passive euthanasia.

Sometimes an appeal to acts and omissions is used to support cases of passive euthanasia. John Ladd (1979) analyses this distinction in terms of theories of intervention linked with causal theories of action and responsibility, and rightly questions the assumption that omissions cannot in fact be causes, especially in health care contexts, where pathology is frequently due to a lack of something.

John Harris (1985, p. 32) also makes this point when he suggests that, in cases where death results from some action not being taken, a frequent question used to establish causation is why that particular action was not taken or performed? Indeed the concept of negligence is based upon the notion of an individual's responsibility for his omissions as well as his actions, such as failure to provide food, clothing, affection, medical care etcetera, thereby causing harm.

As was argued in Chapter 4, it may be appropriate that omissions are viewed as ethically responsible actions as the alternative to provide care and treatment is always available. This is emphasised in clause 2 of the Code of Conduct (UKCC, 1984).

From the foregoing it can be seen that it is far from straightforward to assert that killing is always wrong whereas letting die is always acceptable. If there are moral justifications for any behaviours that result in an individual's death, then they must surely rest on factors other than the particular pigeon-hole into which they fit, or the label that is attached to them.

Indeed, blind acceptance of the differences can lead to morally unacceptable practices such as starving infants to death; cruel, uncaring treatment of patients for fear of killing them; or performing certain actions without question.

Let us now return to consider the classifications relating to consent, in particular, the view that individuals have a right to choose euthanasia.

Voluntary euthanasia

EXIT, the British voluntary euthanasia society, is continually lobbying for euthanasia to become the 'lawful right of the individual, in carefully defined circumstances and with the utmost safeguards, if, and only if, that is his expressed wish' (EXIT, 1980, p. 3). For such exponents, voluntary euthanasia is viewed as an important aspect of human freedom and civil liberty which espouses the belief that autonomous adults should have the freedom to exercise control over their dying as well as their living.

The difficulty lies not in accepting what at first may appear to be a reasonable demand, namely the extension of human freedom, which we might all support, but in determining what constitutes a 'free' or real desire (Lamb, 1988, p. 68).

In Holland, where voluntary euthanasia, although not legalised, is tolerated and openly practised, a code of practice has been established to reassure those involved that all necessary criteria have been satisfied. Such criteria include free will on behalf of the patient; a repeated, deliberate and voluntary request for euthanasia; a consistent wish for death; unacceptable suffering; joint discussion with medical practitioners and nurses involved in the patient's care and with a doctor who is not directly involved with the individual (de Ridder, 1988, pp. 35–6).

In practice, however, such criteria are not at all easy to determine. For example, how are we to ensure that the person is acting under free will? Does the severe pain, fear, or the effect of drugs not affect our ability to make conscious, free and rational decisions? If the person is elderly and has been ill over a long period of time can we be sure that they do not view themselves as a burden on their relatives or carers? Can we be sure that the attitudes of relatives towards the individual concerned have not led to their perceptions of being a nuisance?

Does a repeated wish for death not perhaps represent more of a view about the quality of the care we offer people, rather than a heartfelt desire to end their life? What is to count as unacceptable suffering – years of gnawing, rheumatic pain, mental pain and anguish or intractable pain due to cancer?

In de Ridder's article much emphasis is placed on the opinion of the doctor in establishing these criteria, which may be acceptable if the doctor has good sense, experience and a humane attitude towards his patients. But what if the doctor is inexperienced, lacks sense or is indifferent towards his charges?

An important aspect of voluntariness is the amount of information at our disposal concerning alternative courses of action, and this largely depends on the amount of knowledge that doctors and nurses possess and on their willingness to pass this information on to the patient.

Bearing in mind the pressures on today's health service and the increasing demands for efficiency, it is not beyond the realms of possibility to imagine a scenario where medical staff may be forced into the position of limiting alternative options open to patients because of restricted clinical budgets. In some states in America, referenda are currently being held on euthanasia, no doubt due in part to the worrying escalation of medical costs especially in relation to elderly care and care for AIDS sufferers.

A further point in relation to voluntariness is the notion that having volunteered for something an individual is also free to withdraw, as for example in participating in research studies. Euthanasia does not of course offer this option and the finality of death is one very good reason why we should exercise caution in our consideration of legalising such practices.

Probably the most compelling argument against euthanasia of any sort is the slippery slope or wedge argument. Basically, there are two forms of this argument, the logical version and the empirical version. The logical form focuses on ' . . . how support for one sort of action logically implies support for another sort of action when it is not possible in principle to identify morally relevant dissimilarities' (Beauchamp and Childress, 1983, p. 121). For example, if we approve and accept voluntary euthanasia then there would be no logical way to disapprove of involuntary euthanasia.

Not all philosophers, however, accept this as a valid objection to voluntary euthanasia. James Rachels in refuting supporters of the wedge argument suggests that there are indeed logical or rational differences between an individual who wishes to die because he is in agony and someone who may be old and frail, but who does not wish to die (Rachels, 1986, p. 173).

These differences would include factors such as requests or wishes and the presence of pain or suffering to mention just two. As David Lamb points out, however, this is precisely the warning that is inherent in the logical version of the wedge argument (Lamb, 1988, p. 3). All of the discriminating factors are loose concepts which are therefore prone to disagreement, misinterpretation and misunderstanding. As Lamb states, ' . . . once clear-cut absolutes [i.e. that it is always wrong to kill innocent people] are replaced by intermediate concepts moral boundaries become a playground for sophistry' (Lamb, 1988, p. 4).

The empirical version of the slippery slope argument contends that, once certain procedures or acts are accepted, people will in fact go on to accept other more questionable practices. In other words, it focuses on the ' . . . culture and society to determine the probable impact of changing rules or making exceptions' (Beauchamp and Childress, 1983, p. 122). In the case of voluntary euthanasia, by removing restraints against killing, a general loss of respect for life would result, to the extent that the back door would be opened to non-voluntary and involuntary euthanasia. This is a powerful version of the argument as it is impossible to prove that such results would not in fact happen.

Phillipa Foot, although agreeing that some individual instances of mercy-killing may be right, uses such an argument against changing the law in favour of voluntary euthanasia because of the potential for abuse that would result.

> Many people want, and want very badly, to be rid of their
> elderly relatives and even of their ailing husbands and wives.
> Would any safeguards ever be able to stop them describing as
> euthanasia what was really for their own benefit?
>
> (Foot, 1977, pp. 111–12).

In his response to Foot's concerns, Rachels agrees that, 'there might be some abuses,' indeed he sees the probability of these occurring 'just as there are abuses of virtually every social practice, (Rachels, 1986, p. 175). He does not, however, see this potential as grounds for maintaining the current laws, because the present situation also has its evils and abuses. Instead, he suggests that we should proceed cautiously with reforms.

As Lamb indicates, the present abuses, such as the prolongation of life without reason, are limited naturally by the death of the individual. The abuses forecast by legalising euthanasia would be impossible to contain (Lamb, 1988, p. 5).

One further objection against the legalisation of euthanasia which ought to be addressed is that it is paternalistic and interferes with the individual's liberty. This is certainly a fair criticism, however, weak paternalism is accepted in our society. For example, we have laws enforcing the compulsory education of our children and the taking of various dangerous drugs is prohibited.

In general then, there is a presumption, in our society, that maximising and safeguarding the lives of citizens should, in some situations, override the expression of their autonomy. Voluntary euthanasia is another example of this. As part of the response to this objection, it must also be pointed out that individuals have the right to refuse treatment and the exercise of such a right should not be seen as synonymous with euthanasia, suicide or even a desire to die.

Refusing treatment

If we consider as an example, a Jehovah's Witness who refuses surgery or a blood transfusion for religious reasons, it is quite conceivable that this individual does not wish to die. Indeed, they often pray for divine intervention which would prevent their death.

One of the most famous cases involving the patient's right to refuse treatment was that of Elizabeth Bouvia, a 28-year-old quadriplegic, who was being forcibly fed via a nasogastric tube, while she was a patient in a Californian hospital. The court ruled that 'Being competent, she had the right to live out the remainder of her natural life in dignity and peace' (California Court of Appeal, 1986, p. 1317). The decision caused some confusion for health professionals, some of whom believed that it was authorising passive euthanasia.

This, of course, is not the case for, as long as the doctor or nurse advises of the consequences of discontinuing or refusing treatment and is willing to provide treatment, they cannot be accused of bringing about or contributing in any way to the patient's death.

Further, as we have already seen, a refusal of intervention does not necessarily amount to a desire to die, merely a desire not to be interfered with. Of course this can often place those caring for the individual in a difficult position, not least the nurse whose contact with patients is often more continuous and closer than that of any other health professional.

The nurse may feel that she has failed by not persuading her patient to accept treatment and may feel helpless in a situation that necessitates standing by and watching someone die. As Michael Bayles indicates, this is possibly one of the most difficult issues in nursing ethics ' . . . for it poses the conflict between the nurses' personal values and goals and the responsibilities of being a professional nurse' (Bayles, 1980, p. 2230).

A further problem also exists when, for whatever reason, the person is unable to refuse treatment as for example, when unconscious. In America, public fears that life would be prolonged unduly have resulted in the increasing popularity of 'living wills'. These are written statements, usually made when an individual is well, confirming that they do not wish to undergo life-prolonging treatment should they develop a condition which would result in an impoverished quality of life.

The legal status of these documents is questionable and there have been cases when patients in possession of living wills have been tirelessly resuscitated, to the disgust of their relatives and friends (Schucking, 1985, pp. 261–8).

To overcome these problems many states have enacted what are termed 'Natural Death Acts'. These are directives to doctors to withdraw life-prolonging procedures which serve only to prolong dying, rather than prevent death. In other words, they are only used by patients diagnosed as being terminally ill.

These documents also have their problems in practical usage. For example, many categories of patients are excluded, such as pregnant women, children, those in persistent coma, and the mentally impaired.

This should serve as a warning of the problems that arise when attempting to legislate in an area that is as fraught with difficulties and ambiguities as death is.

The cases

Who decides?

❛ She seemed to be pleading with her eyes for the torment to end ❜

Mrs Evans was a 65-year-old woman who had had surgery for oesophageal carcinoma. In the recovery room Mrs Evans went into respiratory failure following which she was admitted to the intensive care unit and was artificially ventilated.

After two weeks, it was evident that Mrs Evans' condition was unlikely to improve. She had two chest drains inserted for a pneumohaemothorax, her wound was breaking down and she developed crepitus secondary to the assisted ventilation. The doctors believed that this would eventually bring about her death, as it could not be prevented.

Throughout her illness her family were supportive and caring, but they became very distressed at seeing their mother oedematous and in such obvious pain and discomfort. They requested without success that treatment be discontinued. Mrs Evans herself was fully aware and would grimace in pain despite regular analgesia. On two occasions she had tried to extubate herself which had resulted in the doctor ordering arm restraints.

I regularly cared for Mrs Evans, and had discussed with sister my feelings about the continued use of life-support. In fairness sister had also requested that the artificial ventilation be discontinued, and that Mrs Evans be allowed to die peacefully and with dignity, but the medical staff had refused.

One evening the unit was particularly busy and I frequently had to leave Mrs Evans' cubicle to help with other patients. Mrs Evans appeared to be more distressed than ever that evening, despite frequent analgesia, her face was contorted in pain and she seemed to be pleading with her eyes for the torment to end.

Instead of securely fastening the arm restraints, I left them loose enough for Mrs Evans to remove her hand. After a little while the emergency buzzer went in one of the other cubicles. I left Mrs Evans to assist with the patient who had arrested.

On my return I discovered that Mrs Evans had disconnected herself from the ventilator and had died.

No-one ever discovered that my carelessness was deliberate and I felt that my ticking off from the doctor, to be more careful in future, was well worth it as I had acted in Mrs Evans' interest and she was now at peace.

Commentary

This is a particularly difficult case which raises a number of issues. Discussion with colleagues as to the appropriateness of this staff nurse's actions produced much debate as to whether she had behaved courageously, by recognising that her first duty was to act in her patient's best interests or whether in fact she had been unprofessional by assisting her patient to take her own life?

It certainly appears that the patient was unhappy with her situation as she had previously tried to extubate herself. She was in pain and becoming progressively more oedematous as a result of treatment.

We need to ask if the duty to preserve life can justify the imposition of treatment which renders the patient impotent to object. Earlier in the chapter, we noted that all patients have a right to refuse or withdraw from a course of treatment and denial of that right is tantamount to assault. Mrs Evans, because she is unable to speak, is unable to claim that right but that in no way reduces her claim to it.

The staff nurse could perhaps have done more to assist Mrs Evans to express her desire by encouraging the support of her relatives or perhaps even helping her to write down her wishes for treatment to be discontinued. In this way she would have been spared criticism and perhaps, had her actions been discovered, allegations of unprofessional conduct.

We have already discussed advocacy and some of the problems that this poses for the nurse. Suffice it to say that in the light of insufficient guidance as to how to incorporate such responsibilities into the nurse's professional role, the staff nurse could have justifiably claimed that she was in fact acting as patient advocate by supporting her client in the exercise of her autonomy. The UKCC's document *Exericising Accountability* states that 'Each practitioner must determine exactly how this aspect of personal professional accountability is satisfied within her particular sphere of practice' (UKCC, 1989, p. 12).

What of the criticism that the staff nurse assisted the patient in committing suicide? Had the nurse removed Mrs Evans from the ventilator or had she helped her to die by offering an overdose of drugs such an allegation would be well founded. In fact, the nurse merely freed the patient from what appears to have been an unjustified restraint. Mrs Evans chose to use her freedom to detach herself from the ventilator and thereby ended her own life.

What perhaps is most distressing about this case, is that it highlights the urgent need for meaningful dialogue between medical and nursing staff about how best to proceed with the care of particular patients. Although in this example we have only the nurse's views, it would appear that despite the relatives' and other nurses' expressions of disquiet about the prolonged treatment, the doctors were reluctant to discuss any alternatives.

The result in this case is that the nurse feels the need to use subterfuge to best serve Mrs Evans and this could have resulted in feelings of guilt or worse, allegations of misconduct against the nurse, who for the most part, appears to be caring and concerned for the wellbeing of her patients.

A lonely death

❛ I vowed that I would never again allow a patient to die on his own ❜

As a first year student, I remember being dismayed by the attitudes of many of the trained nurses. Most of them found the idea of death distasteful or fearful, and seemed to avoid any contact with dying patients whenever possible.

On one ward there was a 59-year-old man who was dying of congestive cardiac failure. He was a large man who had a great deal of dignity and every day he battled to retain at least a trace of it. The ward itself was a very busy acute elderly care ward with the majority of patients being over 70 years of age.

This man was fully aware and I think he would have received much better care on a medical ward. As the days went by his condition worsened and he was finally moved from the six-bedded area to a side-ward.

To me this meant that he would receive more care and attention and that his special needs would be better met. In reality however it meant that he was merely shut out of the way. No one spent any time even trying to meet his emotional needs and his physical care was in my opinion always hurried and compromised as other patients demanded attention.

I used to try to give him as much care and attention as possible, combing his hair and making sure that he was shaved and felt comfortable. I would tidy his room and open his windows which made him feel better. Before going off duty I would always make sure he had a fresh drink that he could reach and wasn't in need of anything.

On his last morning I was assisting the staff nurse with the medication round. I entered the side-ward to take the patient his drugs and I shall never forget the look on the poor man's face – he was so frightened and fighting for every breath. I am sure he knew that he was going to die. After finishing the medicine round I asked the staff nurse if I could go and sit with him.

She looked at me in disbelief and snapped that 'we don't have time for that sort of thing', as if I were a school child.

My patient died that morning, he was alone, unwashed, his room was a shambles and he had no source of comfort or loving care. Although I am now qualified, the feelings of guilt have never left me although I vowed that day, that regardless of the consequences, never again would I allow a patient to die on their own.

Commentary

This case, unlike the first, does not involve the drama of intensive care units and 'high-tech' machinery. Instead, it involves the care that ought to be available to anyone that is near death, especially when the death is expected and takes place in a hospital, where one of the staff's major concerns should be with the provision of comfort and compassion.

What the case does highlight is the tension that often exists in acute clinical areas between meeting the demands of caring for often seriously ill people, who have a good chance of recovery, and meeting the emotional and spiritual needs of the dying person. These tensions are often made worse by acute staff shortages and lack of resources especially in elderly care areas, not to mention our cultural approach to death.

This student quickly recognised a common criticism of nursing staff, that they regularly avoid contact with dying patients for a variety of reasons. As previously discussed (Chapter 4), one reason often cited is the fact that the truth is frequently withheld from the terminally ill, thus straining relationships to the extent that avoidance is seen as a method of coping with an unsatisfactory situation.

Another factor, however, which may account for these attitudes, is that to a large extent frank discussion about death is taboo in our culture. We find it embarrassing to discuss the possibility of death; as a nation our grieving is largely private and restrained in comparison with some other cultures; and often it is felt to be inappropriate to explore the subject of death with young people.

If programmes of nurse education do not offer the opportunity for students to clarify and come to terms with their own values in relation to death, then it is unlikely that as nurses they will be able to care effectively for terminally ill patients. How are students to learn how to talk with dying patients and discuss death openly if they never observe skilled, qualified practitioners fulfil this vital function?

We need to address the issue of ordering priorities in situations such as the one outlined in this case. It seems fairly obvious that if someone is as close to death as this person so clearly was, then providing companionship and comfort should have come much higher on the staff nurse's list of priorities than it did. After all, it could be argued that one only has one opportunity to meet the needs of someone about to die, whereas all the other tasks to be completed could have been postponed.

The lack of care shown to this patient appears to have had a profound effect on the student, to the extent that she sees it as a priority to offer better care to dying patients. This has, however, been at the cost of experiencing years of guilt which is totally unnecessary and something to be deplored. Perhaps it is examples of such poor and inadequate care that make voluntary euthanasia so desirable an alternative for some people.

Orders for resuscitation

> ❝I felt that . . . she should have been left in peace with her dignity intact❞

During my last year of training, I was working on a medical ward, to which had been admitted a 63-year-old woman in the terminal stages of chest disease. She was a very 'heavy' patient to nurse because of the intensity of the care that she required, but she was always very caring and appreciative towards the nursing staff. She had no family of her own and I think this was one of the reasons why she was so grateful to the staff.

About six days after her admission the consultant and senior registrar were conducting a ward round. As her response to treatment had been so poor and she was obviously becoming weaker, sister asked whether the woman should be resuscitated should she suffer a cardiac arrest. The consultant replied that he would give the matter some thought and let sister know.

Four days later I was working on a late duty along with sister, a staff nurse and an auxiliary nurse. No decision had been recorded about the lady's resuscitation status. Just before supper the patient had been quiet and comfortable but when I went to her after supper I found her in a collapsed state. I felt that I had no choice other than to pull the emergency bell and commence resuscitation although I felt strongly that because of her condition, she should have been left in peace with her dignity intact.

For almost an hour the doctors worked mercilessly on this woman's body and not surprisingly failed to resuscitate her. By the end of the chaos, I almost wished I had pretended not to have found her until it was too late, but I feel it is wrong that nurses should be left in such a position. Doctors should be prepared to make a clear statement when patients are in this situation. On many occasions when this dilemma has arisen, some senior nurses have said we should walk slowly. I've even been told to do this by a junior houseman but I think it is far better to be honest and open about the need to make this type of decision.

Commentary

Many nurses complain about the reluctance of medical colleagues to make decisions about the correct procedures in the case of cardiac arrest, especially with the chronically ill patient.

This leaves nurses in a very vulnerable position for if they ignore the patient and pretend that they have not noticed, then they are open to accusations of negligence and yet they are often acutely aware that the patient has come to terms with death and would prefer not to be subjected to repeated resuscitation. Indeed, it is this tendency to resuscitate everyone that has led to the popularity of living wills and natural death acts in the USA, although as yet they are not commonplace in the UK.

In this country, patients are less likely to be involved in decision-making regarding resuscitation than in America, where the patient is much more likely to be better informed and asked for his opinion. In part, this is probably due to the greater use of litigation in America when individuals are dissatisfied with the health care that either they or their family members receive. But it must be recognised as well that American culture is very much grounded in the theory of rights and this applies as much to the notion that man has a right to retain power over his own death, as it does to any other aspect of his life.

This case highlights quite clearly how, even though the doctors appear to have found some difficulty in making a decision, neither the patient nor the nursing staff are consulted. It could be argued that such decision-making is not properly located within the realms of clinical judgement. Rather it is an ethical decision which affects the individual patient and therefore should primarily take account of his or her beliefs and values.

Preserving and prolonging life are fundamental goals of health care but they are not the only ones. In the case of those near to death, the relief of symptoms and the preservation of independence and dignity should perhaps be the preferred alternatives.

The primary purpose of cardiopulmonary resuscitation is the prevention of sudden, unexpected death, not the prolongation and mechanisation of dying. Only when hospitals develop clear policies relating to resuscitation will such abuses be prevented.

Conclusion

Of all the health professionals involved in patient care, it is frequently the nurse who is most intimately involved with the dying patient and his family. At first, it appears that many of the issues we have discussed primarily affect doctors, such as debates about killing and letting die or decisions regarding resuscitation. However, by virtue of her role, the nurse is also affected by the results of such deliberations.

It is the nursing staff who are left to interpret doctors' orders and to provide care for the patients concerned. Often the nurse's or the patient's beliefs and values are in direct conflict with the decisions taken by medical staff and this can significantly affect the quality of care received by the dying person and their relatives.

One of the emergent themes from each of the cases discussed is the issue of autonomy in the context of feeling in control over one's death and clearly as this is such an important issue for so many people, health care professionals generally, and nurses and doctors in particular, need to take special account of such values.

Because we have no second chances to 'get it right', it is extremely important that nurses use moral reasoning in this area of practice which has perhaps traditionally been the subject of intuitive and emotive responses.

References

Aristotle (1980) *The Nicomachean Ethics*, D. Ross (transl.) (Oxford: Oxford University Press).

Bayles, M. D. (1980) 'The Value of Life – By What Standard?, *American Journal of Nursing*, Dec., pp. 2226–30.

Bayles, M. D. (1983) 'Quality of Life and Euthanasia', in M. D. Bayles and D. High (eds), *Medical Treatment of the Dying*, (Cambridge, Mass: Shenkman Publishing Co.).

Beauchamp, J. M. (1975) 'Euthanasia and the Nurse Practitioner', *Nursing Forum*, vol. XIV, no. 1, pp. 56–73.

Beauchamp, T. L. and Childress, J. F. (1983) *Principles of Biomedical Ethics*, 2nd ed. (New York: Oxford University Press).

California Courts of Appeal Report, 24 April, (1986).

Caroline, N. L. (1972) 'Dying in Academe', *The New Physician*, Nov., pp. 655–7.

de Ridder, C. (1988) 'A Model For Euthanasia', *Nursing Standard*, vol. 3, no. 48, pp. 35–7.

EXIT (1980) *The Last Right: The Need for Voluntary Euthanasia* (London: EXIT).

Foot, P. (1977) 'Euthanasia', *Philosophy and Public Affairs*, vol. 6, pp. 111–12.

Glover, J. (1977) *Causing Death and Saving Lives* (Middlesex: Penguin).

Guardian, 8 January 1985.

Harris, J. (1985) *The Value of Life* (London: Routledge & Kegan Paul).

Ladd, J. (1979) *Ethical Issues Relating to Life and Death* (New York: Oxford University Press).

Lamb, D. (1985) *Death, Brain death and Ethics* (Kent: Croom Helm).

Lamb, D (1988) *Down The Slippery Slope: Arguing in Applied Ethics* (Kent: Croom Helm).

McCormick, R. A. (1974) 'To Save or Let Die', *Journal of American Medical Association*, vol. 229, pp. 172–6.

Melia, K. M. (1987) 'Cruel to be Kind', *Nursing Times*, 8 April, pp. 43–5.

Melia, K. M. (1989) *Everyday Nursing Ethics* (Basingstoke: Macmillan).

Nagel, T. (1986) 'Death', in P. Singer (ed.), *Applied Ethics* (New York: Oxford University Press).

Rachels, J. (1986) *The End of Life: Euthanasia and Morality* (Oxford: Oxford University Press).

Ramsey, P. (1970) *The Patient as Person* (New Haven; Yale University Press).

Riga, P. J. (1989) 'The Health Care Professional and the Care of the Dying: The Crisis of AIDS', *Linacre Quarterly*, February, pp. 53–62.

Schaeffer, E. (1978) *Affliction* (New Jersey: Fleming H Revell Company).

Schucking, E. L. (1985) 'Death in a New York Hospital', *Law, Medicine and Health Care*, December, pp. 261–8.

United Kingdom Central Council for Nurses, Midwives and Health Visitors (1984) *Code of Professional Conduct*, 2nd ed. (London: UKCC).

United Kingdom Central Council for Nurses, Midwives and Health Visitors (1989), *Exercising Accountability* (London: UKCC).

Conclusion

We have tried to present a variety of moral problems experienced by nurses in their day-to-day practice, as well as a discussion of the issues which impinge upon them. One recurring theme has been that of individual autonomy and the difficulties that this raises in health care, be it the patient's or the practitioner's autonomy which is under discussion.

For all nurses this is a central issue as it is nurses who, as people, are dealing with people. People, both individually and generally, are deserving of respect. When respect and autonomy are overridden, the potential for human harm and misery is enormous as the individual or group concerned, is treated as something less than a person – an object to be coerced, manipulated or disregarded.

Having read through the text, you will by now be aware that there are no quick or slick answers that will provide a panacea for the often hard decisions that have to be made. As we have seen, for instance, calls to act in the patient's best interests or to act as the patient's advocate are, in themselves, contentious and may be a source of conflict. What we hope however is that nurses will be better placed to consider how they might respond in similar situations, be willing to explore the reasons and values behind the choices they make and be more aware of the possible implications of alternative courses of action.

Difficult and painful situations will not disappear from nursing, indeed over the next decade, they are likely to increase. Such situations often demand swift action which leaves little time for deliberation. By reflecting on the cases and discussions within this book, we hope that nurses will have, to some extent, clarified their moral positions on issues of importance to them personally. In doing so, not only will they be better prepared to defend and justify the stances that they choose to take, but also, they will be more likely to deliver care in a humane, caring manner.

Right answers in ethics are few and far between, wrong ones are devastating for all those concerned. What is important, however, is that as nurses we continually question our practice.

Appendices

Appendix 1

From *Code for Nurses with Interpretive Statements* ©, 1985, American Nurses' Assocation, Kansas City, Mo., USA (reprinted with permission).

1. The nurse provides services with respect for human dignity and the uniqueness of the client, unrestricted by considerations of social or economic status, personal attributes, or the nature of health problems.
2. The nurse safeguards the client's right to privacy by judiciously protecting information of a confidential nature.
3. The nurse acts to safeguard the client and the public when health care and safety are affected by the incompetent, unethical, or illegal practice of any person.
4. The nurse assumes responsibility and accountability for individual nursing judgments and actions.
5. The nurse maintains competence in nursing.
6. The nurse exercises informed judgment and uses individual competence and qualifications as criteria in seeking consultation, accepting responsibilities, and delegating nursing activities to others.
7. The nurse participates in activities that contribute to the ongoing development of the profession's body of knowledge.
8. The nurse participates in the profession's efforts to implement and improve standards of nursing.
9. The nurse participates in the profession's efforts to establish and maintain conditions of employment conducive to high quality nursing care.
10. The nurse participates in the profession's effort to protect the public from misinformation and misrepresentation and to maintain the integrity of nursing.
11. The nurse collaborates with members of the health professions and other citizens in promoting community and national efforts to meet the health needs of the public.

Appendix 2

Code For Nurses

Ethical concepts applied to nursing, 1973, International Council for Nurses, Geneva (reprinted with permission).

The fundamental responsibility of the nurse is fourfold: to promote health, to prevent illness, to restore health and to alleviate suffering.

The need for nursing is universal. Inherent in nursing is respect for life, dignity and rights of man. It is unrestricted by considerations of nationality, race, creed, colour, age, sex, politics or social status.

Nurses render health services to the individual, the family and the community and coordinate their services with those of related groups.

Nurses and people

The nurse's primary responsibility is to those who require nursing care.

The nurse, in providing care, promotes an environment in which the values, customs and spiritual beliefs of the individual are respected.

The nurse holds in confidence personal information and uses judgement in sharing this information.

Nurses and practice

The nurse carries personal responsibility for nursing practice and for maintaining competence by continual learning.

The nurse maintains the highest standards of nursing care possible within the reality of a specific situation.

The nurse uses judgement in relation to individual competence when accepting and delegating responsibilities.

The nurse when acting in a professional capacity should at all times maintain standards of personal conduct which reflect credit upon the profession.

Nurses and society

The nurse shares with other citizens the responsibility for initiating and supporting action to meet the health and social needs of the public.

Nurses and co-workers

The nurse sustains a cooperative relationship with co-workers in nursing and other fields.

The nurse takes appropriate action to safeguard the individual when his care is endangered by a co-worker or any other person.

Nurses and the profession

The nurse plays the major role in determining and implementing desirable standards of nursing practice and nursing education.

The nurse is active in developing a core of professional knowledge.

The nurse, acting through the professional organisation, participates in establishing and maintaining equitable social and economic working conditions in nursing.

Appendix 3

Code of Professional Conduct for the Nurse, Midwife and Health Visitor, 1984, London (reprinted with permission). United Kingdom Central Council for Nursing, Midwifery and Health Visiting.

Each registered nurse, midwife and health visitor shall act, at all times, in such a manner as to justify public trust and confidence, to uphold and enhance the good standing and reputation of the profession, to serve the interests of society, and above all to safeguard the interests of individual patients and clients.

Each registered nurse, midwife and health visitor is accountable for his or her practice, and, in the exercise of professional accountability shall:

1. Act always in such a way as to promote and safeguard the wellbeing and interests of patients/clients.
2. Ensure that no action or omission on his/her part or within his/her sphere of influence is detrimental to the condition or safety of patients/clients.
3. Take every reasonable opportunity to maintain and improve professional knowledge and competence.
4. Acknowledge any limitations of competence and refuse in such cases to accept delegated functions without first having received instruction in regard to those functions and having been assessed as competent.
5. Work in a collaborative and cooperative manner with other health care professionals and recognise and respect their particular contributions within the health care team.
6. Take account of the customs, values and spiritual beliefs of patients/clients.
7. Make known to an appropriate person or authority any conscientious objection which may be relevant to professional practice.
8. Avoid any abuse of the privileged relationship which exists with patients/clients and of the privileged access allowed to their property, residence or workplace.
9. Respect confidential information obtained in the course of professional practice and refrain from disclosing such information without the consent of the patient/client, or a person entitled to act on his/her behalf, except where

disclosure is required by law or by the order of a court or is necessary in the public interest.

10. Have regard to the environment of care and its physical, psychological and social effects on patients/clients and also to the adequacy of resources, and make known to appropriate persons or authorities any circumstances which could place patients/clients in jeopardy or which militate against safe standards of practice.

11. Have regard to the workload of and the pressures on professional colleagues and subordinates and take appropriate action if these are seen to be such as to constitute abuse of the individual practitioner and/or to jeopardise safe standards of practice.

12. In the context of the individual's own knowledge, experience and sphere of authority, assist peers and subordinates to develop professional competence in accordance with their needs.

13. Refuse to accept any gift, favour or hospitality which might be interpreted as seeking to exert undue influence to obtain preferential consideration.

14. Avoid the use of professional qualifications in the promotion of commercial products in order not to compromise the independence of professional judgement on which patients/clients rely.

Glossary

Acts and omissions doctrine: the view that it is less bad, morally speaking, to bring about a harm by an omission rather than by a positive act, eg., that it is preferable to bring about a person's death by failing to treat rather than by administering a lethal drug.

Altruism: action the aim of which is to benefit one or more people other than the agent.

Autonomy: the capacity for autonomy is the capacity for making choices about one's own life. The principle of autonomy states that those choices should be respected (contrast **paternalism**).

Beneficence: doing good; acting to promote people's interests (compare non-maleficence).

Consequentialism: the name given to types of ethical theory that judge what is right in terms of the consequences, or expected consequences, of actions. The most well-known of these is utilitarianism.

De Facto: as a matter of fact. To say that a person has de facto authority means that people as a matter of fact accept what she says, even if she has no de jure authority.

De Jure: by right. A person who has de jure authority has it as a result of a recognised procedure for placing her in a position of authority, such as an election or a job selection process.

Deontological ethics: the name given to ethical views which state that certain things must be done, or that certain rules or principles must be followed, without considering whether this will lead to the best consequences in particular circumstances.

Ethics: as a subject of study, this may be divided into descriptive, normative and meta-ethics. Descriptive ethics is concerned with what moral views people actually have eg., what nurses think about abortion; normative ethics is concerned with theories as to how to resolve moral dilemmas eg., utilitarianism, which may be applied to the abortion issue; meta-ethics is concerned with the meaning of moral terms eg., if we say that abortion is wrong what does that mean? In this volume we are looking at the application of normative theories to particular cases.

Harm principle: this holds that it is justifiable to override a person's autonomous choice, not for their own good (contrast paternalism), but to prevent them from harming others. The harm to them, of interference, has to be weighed against the harm they might do to others.

Morality: the name given to the device for coping with the problems that arise in areas of life where the interests of different people (or other bearers of interests, such as animals) conflict. It may consist, for example, of a set of principles concerning people's rights or interests. Such principles are the subject-matter of Ethics (*see* **Ethics**).

Non-maleficence: the avoidance of harm to the interests of others (compare **beneficence**).

Normalisation: the current underlying philosophy of mental handicap care defined by Wolfensburger, in 1980, as a process involving the use of culturally valued means in order to enable people to live culturally valued lives.

Paternalism: the overriding of someone's autonomy for what is considered to be their own good eg., not accepting a person's refusal of treatment, on the grounds that it is not in their interests to do so.

Respect for persons: the principle of respect for persons is variously interpreted. It is sometimes used to contrast the treatment appropriate for human beings with that thought appropriate for material things and non-human living organisms: hence the Kantian claim that human beings should be treated as ends in themselves, not as means only. In this volume the principle is taken to involve at least the recognition that human persons have points of view and interests of their own, which should be taken into consideration in deciding how to act.

Rights: a right may be understood as a justified claim to have, receive, or do something eg., the right to have a child, the right to receive treatment, or the right to choose. The success of a rights claim depends on how it is justified. Some take the view that certain rights are self-evident, but in the absence of agreement on this it seems clear that rights have to be argued for. The success of a rights claim will depend on the argument by which it is justified.

Sanctity of life: the principle of the sanctity of life, commonly applied only to human life, is normally taken to mean that human life is valuable for its own sake and that it is wrong deliberately to terminate it.

Slippery slope argument: a type of argument which opposes one action or state of affairs A, because of the danger that it might lead to something worse, B, either because the agent or others will be psychologically 'softened up' by their acceptance of A or because it would be illogical to refuse to accept B if A has been accepted.

Utilitarianism: the ethical theory that states that the right action is what will produce the greatest happiness of the greatest number.

Virtue ethics: a type of ethics which suggests that agents should develop certain character traits, rather than simply following rules or principles.

Suggestions for further reading

Beauchamp, T. L. and Childress, J. F. (1989) *Principles of Biomedical Ethics*, 3rd edn (New York: Oxford University Press).
Dworkin, G. (1988) *The Theory and Practice of Autonomy* (Cambridge: Cambridge University Press).
Gillett, G. (1989) *Reasonable Care* (Bristol: Bristol Press).
Gillon, R. (1985) *Philosophical Medical Ethics* (Chichester: John Wiley).
Glover, J. (1977) *Causing Death and Saving Lives* (Harmondsworth: Penguin).
Harris, J. (1985) *The Value of Life: An Introduction to Medical Ethics* (London: Routledge & Kegan Paul).
Lamb, D. (1988) *Down the Slippery Slope: Arguing in Applied Ethics* (London: Croom Helm).
Lindley, R. (1986) *Autonomy* (Basingstoke: Macmillan).
Lockwood, M. (ed.) (1985) *Moral Dilemmas in Modern Medicine* (Oxford: Oxford University Press).
Raphael, D. D. (1981) *Moral Philosophy* (Oxford: Oxford University Press).
Seedhouse, D. (1988) *Ethics: The Heart of Health Care* (Chichester: John Wiley).
Singer, P. (1979) *Practical Ethics* (Cambridge: Cambridge University Press).

Index